OXFORD MEDICAL PUBLICATIONS

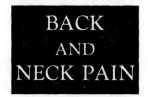

the**facts**

D1246432

the**facts**
ALSO AVAILABLE IN THE SERIES

BACK AND NECK PAIN

thefacts

Loïc Burn

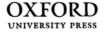

OXFORD
UNIVERSITY PRESS

*This book has been printed digitally and produced in a standard specification
in order to ensure its continuing availability*

OXFORD
UNIVERSITY PRESS

Great Clarendon Street, Oxford OX2 6DP

Oxford University Press is a department of the University of Oxford.
It furthers the University's objective of excellence in research, scholarship,
and education by publishing worldwide in

Oxford New York

Auckland   Cape Town Dar es Salaam Hong Kong Karachi
Kuala Lumpur Madrid Melbourne Mexico City   Nairobi
New Delhi Shanghai Taipei Toronto
With offices in
Argentina Austria Brazil Chile Czech Republic France Greece
Guatemala Hungary Italy Japan South Korea Poland Portugal
Singapore Switzerland Thailand Turkey Ukraine Vietnam

Oxford is a registered trade mark of Oxford University Press
in the UK and in certain other countries

Published in the United States
by Oxford University Press Inc., New York

© Loic Burn, 2000

ISBN 0-19-263077-6

the**facts**

CONTENTS

1
Introduction

When someone has a medical problem they ask four main questions. What IS it? What will it DO to me? What will THEY (the clinicians) do to me? What can I (self-help) do about it? Back and neck pain raises some additional complications. Firstly, for unknown reasons, it is a neglected subject in medical education. This means that your doctor is likely to be less informed about it than about other common conditions. Secondly, there are specific problems in making an accurate diagnosis (which we cover in some detail later). Thirdly, and probably as a result of the first two, there are many different groups all offering you various treatments and advice—much more so than for other medical problems. This may be very confusing for you and in this book we try to provide a balanced view of everything that is on offer. However, there are few areas where actually more information for patients is needed.

Happily there have been two recent changes that have altered the situation to your advantage.

Firstly, the National Back Pain Association (NBPA) runs a helpline for people who suffer with back pain. Myrad Kinloch of Kingston University did an analysis of the queries received by the helpline and we now have a clearer picture of the many different ways in which back and neck pain could affect your life (what it will do to you). It also tells us of your commonest concerns and worries. With this knowledge we are now better able to address directly your actual needs.

Secondly, and much more importantly, the scale of the problem in all developed countries is so great and growing so fast that governments—especially here, in Sweden, and in the USA—have felt compelled to take action. The USA in particular has undertaken an enormous amount of research in recent years which has revolutionized diagnosis (what IS it), management (what THEY do), and self-help (what YOU do). The Clinical Standards Advisory Group (CSAG) published a report on the management of back pain using much of this new evidence. This was sympathetically received by the government. In September 1996 the Royal College of General Practitioners (RCGP) published further management guidelines, very much in line with the report, based on evidence obtained between April 1994 and April 1996. So fast are things moving that a further review was undertaken in April 1998 based on the work done up until then. These impressive advances have all worked, as we will show, to your advantage. They have made some previous knowledge obsolete and proved some to be incorrect. Better results are likely if you are fully aware of what is going on and use that information to work positively with your clinician.

Finally, neck pain is a more neglected medical area than back pain; it is less common and there is very little published on it. People who suffer from neck pain may, therefore, feel even more isolated than those who suffer from back pain. There are many similarities between neck and back pain, and these we detail. Where there are differences we devote special sections to self-help for acute and chronic neck pain and to specific queries on neck pain received by the NBPA helpline. We hope that those people who suffer from neck pain will get just as much out of this book as those who suffer from back pain.

Objectives

1. We discuss the causes and extent of the problem.
2. We deal with the diagnosis of your back and neck pain: the new guidelines from the CSAG .
3. We assess your experience of acute (short-lived) pain, your management of it, the new CSAG guidelines, and self-help.
4. We do the same for chronic (long-standing) pain.
5. We detail the various people who may help you and the treatments they may offer.
6. We show how you can get the most out of your consultations.

7. We review your most common back and neck pain queries and provide answers to frequently asked questions.

8. We integrate neck pain into this general scenario.

2 How your back and neck are built and work

Before discussing the huge and growing problem of back and neck pain it is essential to have some idea of how the whole system is built and works. We will show you what an extraordinarily complicated structure it is. This may help you to appreciate some of the problems clinicians face when trying to make an accurate diagnosis. We will also demonstrate how some positions put you at greater risk of developing pain, and how if specific neck structures are damaged, manipulation can be dangerous.

Objectives

1. We discuss the vertebrae, the intervertebral disc, and the posterior vertebral joints.
2. We describe the spinal canal and cord.
3. We review the ligaments, tendons, and muscles.
4. We comment on the vertebral arteries.

1. The vertebrae, the intervertebral disc, and the posterior vertebral joints

The vertebrae

Between your skull and pelvis there are twenty-four bones—the vertebrae. These are in three groups: five cervical (neck) vertebrae, twelve thoracic (middle back) vertebrae, and five lumbar (lower back) vertebrae. This column 'stands' on your sacrum (a triangular bone at the back of the pelvis made up of five fused vertebrae) and the coccyx (a rudimentary 'tail' made up of fused vertebrae at the base of the spine). This is shown in Figure 1. The vertebrae that take the greatest strain of physical activity are in the lumbar region, which may be why low-back pain is so common. Although in reality your whole spine is involved to some extent in every movement, for our purposes it is convenient to think of movements as taking place between just two neighbouring vertebrae known as the mobile segment. This can be seen in Figure 2. All the structures in the mobile segment have to move at the same time. Moreover it is impossible for just one to move at any time—bits of your back never work in isolation, they all work together.

All your vertebrae have a common structural plan. This includes a vertebral body in front and a number of bony outgrowths (the pedicles; the laminae; and the articular, spinous, and transverse processes). These are shown in Figure 3. (There are, however, some important variations on this common plan which we will discuss later.) When

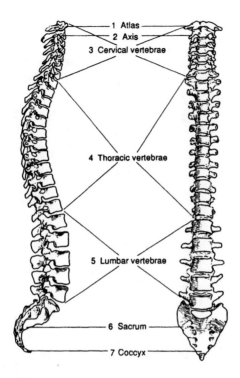

Figure 1

you are sitting or standing, the vertebral bodies are the main weight-bearing elements of your spine. Because of their size, shape, and arrangement they play a part in both allowing and limiting movement (see Figure 2). The spinous and transverse processes act as levers, to which muscles are attached by their tendons (see tendons) and through which the muscles pull and relax when you move or maintain your posture. Any movement requires some muscles to pull, while others relax. If all muscles pulled

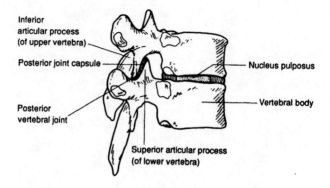

Inferior
articular process
(of upper vertebra)

Posterior joint capsule

Posterior
vertebral joint

Superior articular process
(of lower vertebra)

Nucleus pulposus

Vertebral body

Figure 2

together your spine would stiffen and movement
would be prevented.

The intervertebral disc

Any two vertebrae (save for the first two cervical
vertebrae) are joined together in front by the

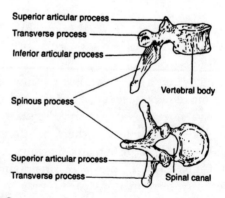

Superior articular process

Transverse process

Inferior articular process

Spinous process

Vertebral body

Superior articular process

Transverse process

Spinal canal

Figure 3

intervertebral disc and behind by a pair of small joints—the posterior vertebral joints (sometimes known as the zygo-apophyseal joints). See Figure 4.

The intervertebral disc consists of a tough, slightly elastic ring called the annulus fibrosus. This is made in layers, its oblique fibres going alternately one way or the other. The annulus fibrosus is very firmly attached to the edges of the vertebral bodies above and below, and also to the thin cartilaginous end-plates of the vertebral bodies. The annulus fibrosus ring contains a jelly-like substance, the nucleus pulposus, and plays a part in spinal movement. This is shown in Figure 5.

When you think how heavy the upper part of your body is you can imagine how extreme the forces are in your lower spine. If these forces are too great or too sudden you are in danger of damaging your back.

Any pressure placed on a mobile segment will distort the elastic annulus fibrosus of the disc and

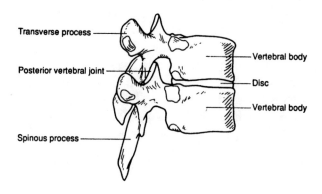

Transverse process

Vertebral body

Posterior vertebral joint

Disc

Vertebral body

Spinous process

Figure 4

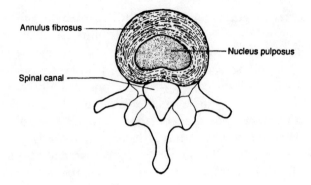

Annulus fibrosus

Nucleus pulposus

Spinal canal

Figure 5

the nucleus pulposus. Because of the way the annulus is built it will stretch in different directions. This allows one vertebra to press down on the next one, or to twist slightly onto its neighbour, or tip it forwards, backwards, or sideways, or it can slide over its neighbour. When you move your back several of these things may happen at the same time and a problem with any of them can cause pain.

Research has thrown much light on pressures within the intervertebral disc. For example, dangerously high pressures in your lower discs and subsequent possible damage to the spine are produced by leaning forward whilst sitting and then picking up a quite modest weight, such as a telephone directory. This has significant practical implications for the working environment. High pressures are also produced by doing exercises that involve bending—including the widely used sit-up! Unfortunately, few fitness coaches are aware of this. If you do take part in fitness or exercise classes it is always worth discussing routines with your doctor; he or she should be able to advise you about whether or not they are safe for your back and neck.

The posterior vertebral joints

These are much smaller than the disc and are in pairs between the articular processes (the touching, sliding surfaces) of neighbouring vertebrae. The surfaces of these joints are lined with cartilage, which is lubricated by joint fluid contained in a joint capsule which, in turn, is supported by a number of small ligaments. This is shown in Figure 6.

The joints take part in weight bearing and also in movement of the mobile segment. During movement the surfaces of these joints may be pushed together, pulled apart, or angled to each other, or they may slide across each other in one direction or another. All this may occur, to

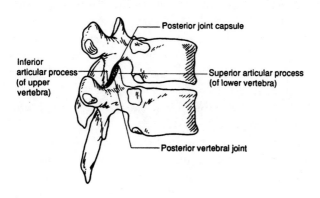

Inferior articular process (of upper vertebra)

Posterior joint capsule

Superior articular process (of lower vertebra)

Posterior vertebral joint

Figure 6

varying degrees, every time you change position. Different strains will therefore be put on different parts of your spine. Pain can occur if anything interferes with the posterior vertebral joints.

2. The spinal canal and cord

As you can see from Figure 3 there is a hole down the middle of the vertebrae—the spinal canal. Between each pair of vertebrae there are two holes running sideways—the lateral canals. The spinal canal contains and protects the spinal cord. The lateral canals protect the nerve roots as they branch out from the spinal cord to the rest of the body.

The spinal cord is made up of nerve material and is an extension of the brain. It is shorter than the spinal canal and only reaches as far as the first lumbar vertebra. It is protected by a sheath called the dura mater. Within the dura mater the spinal cord floats in the cerebrospinal fluid—the same fluid that surrounds your brain. From the spinal cord come pairs of nerves, one pair for each vertebral level, each protected by its own sheath of dura. Because the spinal cord is shorter than the bony structure and ends at the first lumbar vertebra, the lower nerve roots extend quite a distance down the spinal canal before they find their own lateral canals and branch down into the legs. Over this section the nerves are at risk of interference from anything else which might take up space in the spinal canal or the lateral canals. This could include a damaged intervertebral disc. See Figure 7.

3. The ligaments, tendons, and muscles

The ligaments

The whole structure is supported by a system of seven ligaments. They are strong, fibrous and inelastic bands which hold the bones of the skeleton together and add strength to all the joints. These are shown in Figures 8a and 8b.

They not only help to hold the column of vertebrae together, but also help restrict too much movement which might otherwise cause damage. When your back is fully bent forwards, your back muscles play no part in maintaining your position and the ligaments take over. In the neck some of them may be damaged if you have rheumatoid arthritis. If this is the case, manipulation is out of the question, because a damaged ligament may rupture and serious injury may result.

The tendons

These are the ropes which attach your muscles to your bones. Contracting a muscle pulls the tendons, bringing the points of bony attachment nearer together. If there is a joint between the two bones the muscle is attached to, then such a pull will move that joint. It may be stopped from moving if another opposing muscle contracts at the same time, or if there is a physical obstruction to movement. But the muscular pull is always transmitted through your tendons.

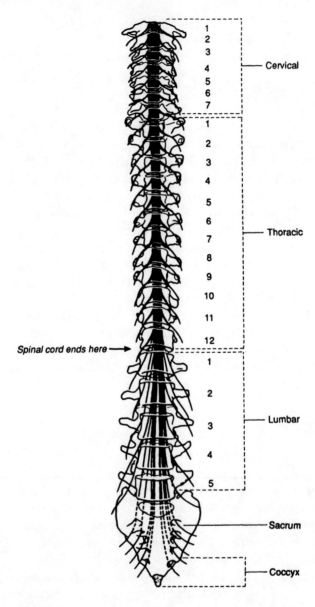

Figure 7

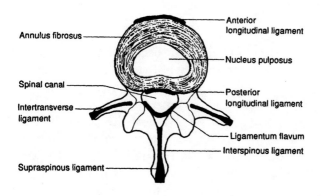

(a)

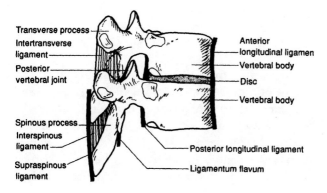

(b)

Figure 8

The muscles

Muscle activity can now be measured and recorded with great accuracy using highly sensitive devices which register tiny changes in the flow of electric current. Muscles either contract or relax their contraction, and they can do this to very slight degrees. There are hundreds of muscles involved in moving your back and neck, and what they do varies so widely that no clinician can be certain what any individual muscle is doing at any one time. Unfortunately, sports and fitness coaches may not be aware of the latest thinking and many exercises are based on outdated ideas as to how muscles work. If you suffer from back or neck pain, but want to maintain your fitness, always ask a doctor to comment on your routines.

4. The vertebral arteries

These, as shown in Figure 9, are important as the source of blood supply to your brain. You will see that each artery kinks before it enters your skull. Some head movements may temporarily block one of these arteries. This has no effect so long as the other one is not restricted. If, on the other hand, you suffer from arterial disease (fairly

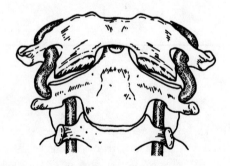

Figure 9

common in older people), both arteries may be restricted. Blockage in one can then cause problems. Treatment for some spinal pain may involve manipulation of the neck. This should not be carried out if you suffer from arterial disease because of the risk and possible fatal consequences of cutting off the blood supply to the brain. So, if you get giddy if you stand up or turn suddenly (a symptom of this disease), manipulation is not for you.

Conclusion

There are about fifty bones, one hundred joints, one thousand muscles, and a million nerves in your back and neck. So it is hardly surprising that back and neck pain are among the most common of physical afflictions. There is so much to go wrong! However, having described the amazing piece of machinery called the back and neck you can now perhaps sympathize with the doctors as they try to trace the source of your pain. In addition, you are armed with some of the information necessary to understand what is happening to you.

Key points

1. The enormous complexity of your back and neck probably makes it impossible to identify specific tissues as the cause of your pain.
2. The spine may be at greater risk when bending forward than when it is straight.

3. To identify individual, problem spinal muscles and strengthen them by exercise is not possible.

4. If you have rheumatoid arthritis of the neck do NOT have your neck manipulated as ligament damage may put your life at risk.

5. The same is true if you have arterial disease and get giddy on standing or turning suddenly.

3

The causes and extent of the problem

Introduction

The causes of back and neck pain have been investigated intensively for many years in the hope of finding ways to prevent them. The outcome of all this work may be both surprising and comforting.

Objectives

1. We look at such causes as evolution, cultural factors, age, gender, association with other complaints, and smoking.
2. We discuss workplace factors, malingering, posture, and 'wear and tear'.
3. We see what this means for the advice you are so frequently given.
4. We review the present 'epidemic' and work loss, particularly with regard to chronic pain.

1. Potential causes

Evolution

One suggestion is that all back and neck trouble is due to the fact that humans have adopted the erect posture. However, since we know that our 'ancestors' were walking upright as long as four million years ago and have evidence of changes, notably in relation to the teeth, that have taken place as a consequence of the human erect posture, it seems inconclusive to blame evolution.

Cultural factors

Another proposed theory for back and neck pain is that in pre-neolithic times the hunter/gatherer undertook probably fifty lifts a day, whereas in the post-industrial revolution era workers could perform up to five thousand lifts a day. However, so many other things have changed (for example, diet) that to isolate a single factor in this way is too simplistic an answer.

Age

This is one area of good news. Most people believe that back and neck troubles steadily increase with the years and that if they start early in life then the inevitable end is a wheelchair. The truth is much more comforting than this. The number of people with back or neck pain rises from the late teens to the early forties and thereafter remains relatively constant. So old age is not synonymous with back pain! There are few pieces of information that patients are happier to hear.

Gender

There is no difference in the frequency of back pain between men and women and very little in relation to the amount of disability and work loss.

Association with other complaints

Back and neck pain are very common complaints. In fact only headache and tiredness are more common. It is perhaps, therefore, not surprising that no 'leads' in this area have been found.

Smoking

In contrast, however, there is much evidence that back pain occurs more frequently in smokers. So here is another incentive to stop smoking!

2. The workplace, malingering, posture, and 'wear and tear'

Work factors

It is generally thought that back pain is more common in people doing heavy manual jobs and those involving heavy lifting. Since not all investigators are convinced of this link however, the most we can say with any certainty is that heavy jobs and those involving heavy vibration may produce increased back pain. We do at least have figures to support the link between heavy lifting and increased back pain for those involved in nursing.

Malingering

There has been much discussion as to the link, if any, between back pain, disability, and early retirement. Many people believe in the connection between back pain and malingering. It is an extremely complicated and contentious subject and, again, there is no agreement and no convincing evidence.

We return to this theme in Chapter 9, as it is one of the major problems you face. In fact, as we show in Chapter 16, being off work is, naturally, a very serious concern and preoccupation for everybody, particularly in the present day.

Posture

'Bad' posture is often cited as a key cause of back pain. In fact, surprisingly, the connection has never been proved. Similarly, fitness has not been shown to reduce the risk of back pain. Also, there is no proven correlation between height or weight and back pain, except in the very tall or obese. So, whilst all these factors have been repeatedly proposed as major causes of back pain, none have ever been confirmed as such.

'Wear and tear'

Another widely held belief, by doctors as well as others, is that ageing is responsible for much backache. We have already seen that this is not the case. Nevertheless, patients are often told that because an X-ray of their spine shows 'wear and tear', this is responsible for their pain. Rest assured, there is no proven relationship between such X-ray changes and spinal pain. As a cause of much unnecessary worry for you, we return to this common but mistaken view in Chapter 15.

3. Advice on prevention

Clinicians may often give conflicting and very dogmatic advice, particularly with regard to such issues as posture. As we have seen, however, there is no conclusive evidence on the causes of back pain. If the advice given to relieve your pain seems to help, then all well and good. But if it does not help, or even makes the pain worse, then challenge your clinician to reconsider. Remember, however, that advice given to reduce the level of disability may involve some pain and discomfort but may ultimately allow you to lead a much more normal life—possibly with less pain as well.

The right advice is not always appreciated: one patient's reaction

A patient had low back pain for twenty-five years. Twenty years ago a clinician informed her that the cause, as for all back pain, was bad posture, and that the solution was to maintain a complicated sitting posture for several hours a day. She had great faith in this advice which she dutifully carried out and which presented only one problem. She found that if she had pain at the beginning of this procedure it invariably worsened towards the end, and if she did not have pain to begin with it was always brought on by this activity. We told her that there was really no such thing as bad posture and it would be sensible to avoid any position that brought on or worsened her pain. She was unhappy with this advice and continued as before, on the grounds that her pain might worsen if she stopped.

4. The effects of back and neck pain on work levels

The 'epidemic'

The scale of the problem of back and neck pain, and its apparently inexorable growth is a matter of great concern for the government. As well as the increasing number of work days being lost (and the economic effect of that), there are also the additional costs of social security payments, strains on NHS resources, and so on.

Loss of work

The increase in time off work shown in Figure 10 is thought to be due to a variety of factors including the changing ideas, attitudes, and expectations of the clinicians and the public. Comparable trends have been noted in other countries. We now know that the number of days off work doubled between 1970 and 1980

Million days p.a.

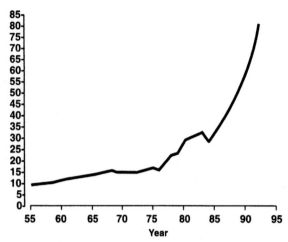

Figure 10 Total British sickness and invalidity benefit for back incapacities

from 15 to 30 million days and doubled again between 1980 and 1990 to 60 million. The latest statistics show that this worrying pattern is likely to be repeated for the current decade (the number of days lost between 1991 and 1992 came to 81 million, and between 1993 and 1994 to 106 million).

Figures 11 and 12 indicate this increase in loss of work in terms of the estimated annual health care costs. A dramatic increase is evident between 1985 and 1993. (Obviously, time off work is only one way of measuring the misery that back and neck pain can cause you. Chapters 9 and 16 look at how they can affect many different aspects of your life.) A summary of the cost of back pain is shown in Figures 13 and 14.

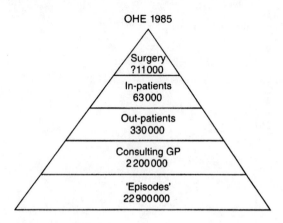

Figure 11 Estimated annual health care for back pain in 1985 (OHE 1985).

The two graphs (Figures 13 and 14) showing the duration of work loss with back pain and the probability of return to work paint a picture

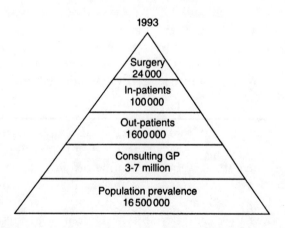

Figure 12 Estimated annual health care for back pain in 1993.

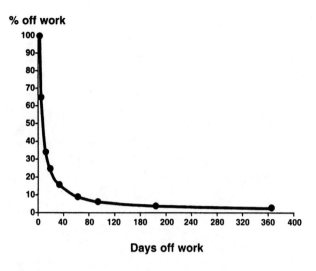

Figure 13   Duration of work loss with back pain.

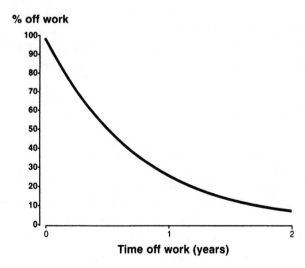

Figure 14   Probability of return to work.

every bit as disturbing—if not more so. They demonstrate that the longer you have been off work, the less likely you are to go back. To reduce the likelihood of this happening the CSAG guidelines insist on early and active treatment. So if your pain lasts more than a few days it is important to get treatment quickly, otherwise the future consequences can be considerable (see Chapters 7 and 8).

Although chronic pain is rather more difficult to deal with than acute (short-lived) pain, people who have had pain for some time have problems which, if identified, can often still be helped (see Chapters 10 and 11).

The neck

There is no evidence of any difference in relation to the causes and risk factors between neck pain and low back pain. The frequency of neck pain is only slightly less than that of low back pain but the consequences are, happily, far less severe.

Conclusion

So, there are few, if any, clear-cut causes to account for the growing back and neck pain 'epidemic'—and 'epidemic' it is. Obviously a major new approach is needed to tackle the problem and this is discussed in Chapters 5, 6, and 10. On the other hand, we are each best placed to find out what suits us best in terms of posture, activity, and so on.

Key points

1. Back and neck pain do not occur more in old age.

2. Apart from smoking, risk factors are uncertain; dogmatic advice on prevention is misplaced.

3. Stop smoking.

4. There has been an explosion in the amount of time off work due to back and neck pain.

5. Because the longer you are off work, the less likely you are to return, a policy of early and active treatment is obviously to your advantage, and you need to ensure that you get it.

6. This does not mean that if you have had back or neck pain for some time that nothing can be done for it. It is simply rather more difficult.

7. The causes and risk factors are the same for both back and neck pain. The scale of the problem in relation to neck pain is smaller but the advice with regard to prevention is identical.

4
Your spinal pain—top to toe

Introduction

There are two important, potentially confusing facts about the spine and pain. Firstly, problems in the spine can, and frequently do, lead to pain felt in almost any part of the body. When such pain is felt at a distance from its true source it is called 'referred' pain. With spinal pain this is very common indeed and, unfortunately, can make the diagnosis difficult. Tenderness can be referred in exactly the same way, and is as unreliable in indicating its source. The problems created by referred pain are discussed in the next chapter.

Objectives

1. We discuss headaches and 'migraines'.
2. We review bizarre symptoms coming from neck and whiplash injuries.

3. We describe referral of neck pain to the shoulder and arm and down the back.
4. We deal with pain referred to the chest and abdomen.
5. We comment on pain referred to the lower back and on 'true' low back pain.

1. Headaches and 'migraines'

It has been claimed that perhaps as many as one out of three headaches originate in the neck. So if you need to see your doctor because you are suffering from frequent headaches, you should ask to have your neck examined. Problems with the neck often cause 'one-sided' headaches which may be misdiagnosed as migraine. Again, if you suffer from these symptoms ask your doctor or another qualified clinician to look at your neck. If the headaches are found to relate to a neck problem, then a variety of local treatments may be of help to you.

2. Bizarre symptoms and whiplash injuries

Bizarre symptoms of spinal origin

These are peculiar symptoms that you might not expect to come from your neck, and may include giddiness and ringing in the ears. They are not uncommon but often confuse doctors because they may suggest ear, nose, and throat (ENT) conditions. A misdiagnosis is possible since the spinal origin of these symptoms is not widely known. If an ENT assessment produces no positive evidence, it is worth asking to see a back and neck specialist.

Whiplash injuries

Headache, and the symptoms just described, may follow whiplash injury (a neck 'sprain' commonly caused by road traffic accidents).

Again, as the connection is not well-known, your neck may not be examined. You may be considered to be neurotic or to be suffering from 'post-traumatic neurosis' if you continue to complain. This is unfortunate because several different treatments applied to the neck might alleviate your pain. If you have aches and pains after an accident or ENT-like symptoms you should again ask to see a specialist. (See Chapter 17.)

3. Referral of pain to the shoulder and arm and the upper back

This is not uncommon with neck problems and it can be a source of confusion. Referred tenderness can produce physical signs which, if the spine is not examined, may indicate a tennis elbow or carpal tunnel syndrome (a condition that causes pain/altered sensations in the hand), when in fact the symptoms are caused by problems in the spine.

Pain between your shoulder blades often originates from your neck. If this is not considered, treatment may well prove unsatisfactory, as it will be targeted on the wrong place.

4. Pain referred to the chest and abdomen

Spinal pain is often referred to the chest—with possible serious consequences. If the spine is not examined this pain may be interpreted as indicating heart disease. In one university hospital in Denmark patients admitted because of acute chest pain were studied over two years. In 20 per cent of them their pain was traced to their spines.

Abdominal pain is not often associated with the spine. However, misdiagnosis can lead to unnecessary abdominal investigations and even to surgery. In one case a patient's abdomen was operated on no fewer than three times, when in fact his problems were spinal.

5. Pain referred to the low back and 'true' low back pain

Again, this is not widely recognized and it is not unusual for patients to receive extensive treatment to the lumbar spine—even surgery—when the pain really arises higher up in the back.

As already stated, low back pain can be referred from other parts of the spine. But it can also arise from the lumbar spine itself. It can be referred from the lumbar spine to the buttocks, coccyx, and to either or both legs.

Conclusion

You can see how spinal pain can indeed be felt from top to toe. More important, it can often lead to misdiagnosis as different as migraine, heart disease, and appendicitis. Whilst not enough doctors are aware of this, training in back problems is improving. However, if you feel that you might fit into one of the scenarios described in this chapter, be prepared to ask your doctor to refer you to a back or neck specialist. Remember that the proper treatment is often highly successful; without it your symptoms are unlikely to improve.

Key points

1. Up to one third of headaches may be caused by neck problems.
2. Migraine is commonly misdiagnosed and may be simply unilateral head pain coming from the neck.
3. Bizarre ENT symptoms may again be coming from the neck.
4. If headaches or bizarre symptoms persist after a whiplash injury the neck may be the cause.
5. Pain from the spine may be referred down the arms and back and present a confusing clinical picture.
6. Spinal pain can be referred to the chest and abdomen and may be interpreted as indicating heart or abdominal conditions.

7. These problems are very common so that if you think that your symptoms 'fit the bill' be prepared to ask to see a back specialist.

8. This is all the more important because if the problem is correctly identified treatments such as manipulation, injection, or acupuncture are usually very effective.

5
Your neck and back pain diagnosis

Introduction

More than for any other medical problem, it is difficult to say what causes neck and back pain and also to define what exactly it is. On the other hand, the CSAG guidelines (see Chapter 1) include a system of case analysis to be used by doctors which greatly clarifies matters not only for them but also for you. This is particularly important with the existence of literally hundreds of confusing diagnostic labels. This chapter explores the issues and, hopefully, reassures you.

Objectives

1. We outline why it is impossible to give a 'true' diagnosis in most cases.
2. We explain what 'numb bum', 'red flags', nerve root pain, and simple neck and back pain

are—and how you can use this knowledge to your advantage.

3. We discuss the issue of diagnostic 'labels' and their implications for your life and the treatment you receive.

4. We describe how you can simplify matters by ignoring such labels.

5. We deal with your neck pain diagnosis.

1. The problem of diagnosis

What is the reason for all the confusion concerning diagnosis? It is because the nerve endings that respond to painful stimuli are present in the majority of tissues that make up your spine and surrounding structures (a large and complicated system, as seen in Chapter 2). In addition, there is the problem of referral which means that pain coming from a spinal tissue can be felt at a distance from its site of origin. For example, pain coming from anywhere in the lower back can be felt anywhere in the leg. Unfortunately, for the purposes of making a diagnosis, it is difficult to tell from where a referred pain is emanating. So, if you have been gardening all day and in the evening you have back or neck pain, who can possibly tell which tissue or tissues it is coming from?

2. The CSAG guidelines for diagnosis

The guidelines suggest a simple and very helpful system of diagnosis for GPs which you yourself may find interesting and useful.

The serious problems

The first task for the doctor is to make sure that the pain is actually coming from the spine because it can be referred from the abdomen or the bladder, or be gynaecological in origin. He or she then has to identify the serious problems that need urgent specialist attention.

The 'numb bum'

The first of these serious problems is luckily, exceedingly rare. If you develop back pain, with or without leg pain, and in addition get a numb bum or problems with your bowel or bladder, you must get in touch with your doctor immediately. The nerve supply to your bladder may be involved and prompt treatment could prevent lifelong bladder problems.

The 'red flags'

As the term suggests, these are urgent medical conditions and include infections of the spine, tumours of various kinds, inflammatory diseases of the joints such as ankylosing spondylitis, and problems involving nerve damage (which may follow an accident such as a fall or a car crash). The pain may be 'non-mechanical', meaning it is constant and progressive and is not related to activity, position, or movement and may be worse at night in bed. Anyone with a previous history of cancer should be looked at carefully if he or she presents with this type of pain. Similar careful screening should apply to anyone who feels unwell in themselves or has recently lost weight or has a persistent and severe restriction of forward bending. Finally, anyone presenting with back or neck pain after the age of 55 has to be thoroughly investigated for 'red flag' conditions.

These then are the conditions requiring urgent attention that doctors are warned to look out for. In total they account for less than one per cent and are relatively easy to identify. If you are in the tiny minority that has them, your doctor will refer you urgently to a specialist, whom you are likely to see within a few weeks. If you have an inflammatory problem, your doctor will probably choose a rheumatologist—if there is one available locally—as they are specially trained in dealing with these problems. If the condition involves serious nerve damage, you will see an orthopaedist or neurosurgeon, as you may have something pressing on a nerve that will require surgical removal.

Nerve root problems

Basically this refers to sciatica, or pain in the leg. (You can have nerve root problems arising from the neck, with pain in the arm—but this is very rare.) The symptoms include pain in one leg, with or without back pain. The pain is typically sharp and clearly localized and is commonly felt below the knee, down to the foot or toes. It may be associated with numbness or tingling in the same area. It is usually caused by a prolapsed intervertebral disc (which means that a part of a disc is pressing on a nerve root), by spinal stenosis (narrowing of the spinal canal), or by surgical scarring (following a back operation). All of these can cause contact with and pressure on a nerve root.

How these problems are treated is described in Chapter 7. The important point is that this group constitutes less than five per cent of all back pain and much less (we don't know precisely how much less) of all neck pain. In other words, a very small percentage. Most cases can also be effectively treated.

Simple backache and neck pain

There is one diagnostic group left to consider— called 'simple'—which comprises 95 per cent of all spinal pain. It is described as 'mechanical' which means that it comes from spinal tissues but is not due to a specific and identifiable disease such as cancer or an inflammatory disease such as, for example, rheumatoid arthritis. Whilst this group includes a multitude of conditions, it has a number of distinguishable features that make identification easier. For example, 'mechanical' pain varies with physical activities such as standing, sitting, and walking. (Contrast this with 'red flag' pain which typically is constant and does not vary at all, neither with activity nor between the morning and the evening.) It usually occurs between the ages of 20 and 55. Additionally, patients feel well in themselves; they don't feel ill (which again is in contrast to those suffering typical 'red flag' pain). Finally, there is a good recovery rate for patients in this group; 90 per cent get better within six weeks. For doctors, this straightforward checklist of features certainly simplifies diagnosis.

Your own diagnostic category

Knowledge of the three diagnostic groups that you can be 'slotted' into can only serve to your advantage. If you have the bad luck to be one of the few to fall into the group of serious problems, you at least know that your problem will be quickly identified and dealt with appropriately. (The hospital consultation, what happens to you, and how to get the most out of the consultation is covered in Chapter 11.) The remaining two groups account for 99 per cent of back and neck pain problems and the majority of cases can and should be handled within the general practice. (What the doctors do to you and what you can do for yourself is described in Chapters 7 and 8.)

Indeed, given the information already provided on symptoms and signs, it would be a relatively simple and reassuring job for you to determine your own diagnostic category. Such information also helps when clinicians insist on using medical jargon. Remember, the CSAG guidelines on diagnosis aim to make the process as straightforward for you as for the clinicians.

3. Diagnostic 'labels'

Even though we know that in most cases a specific diagnosis is not possible, there are still literally hundreds of diagnostic 'labels' that are or have been used including a slipped disc, arthritis, a trapped nerve, lateral canal syndrome, sacro-iliac strain, cervical spondylosis, and so on. Many different groups of people (including doctors), all with their own ideas, and often with their own vocabularies, have, over many decades, contributed to the list. The result is that you are likely to be given different diagnoses from different people for the same set of symptoms and, what is worse, offered widely differing and sometimes contradictory advice by almost as many people as you care to consult—a confusing and worrying situation to say the least. (See Chapter 16.)

Case history: the experience of one patient with back pain

'I have had back pain on and off for about 10 years. Sometimes it lasts longer than a week, and it is so severe that I can't work. One attack lasted more than six weeks. I was very disappointed in my GP. He never examined me and only asked where the pain was and whether I had done anything to bring the pain on. He told me to stay in bed, but that didn't help. Finally he had an X-ray taken and said that it showed a lot of wear and tear and that I had to learn to live with it.

I asked my friends what I should do and got a lot of conflicting advice. In the end I went to an osteopath and he helped me. But the next bad attack that I got did not respond to his treatment or to that of a chiropractor or an acupuncturist that I went to. It finally cleared up on its own. They all told me that my pain was due to different causes which I found very confusing and unsatisfactory, although sometimes their treatment helped.'

4. Your response to the confusion

Sadly, this sort of story is not uncommon. However, such worrying and perplexing confusion can be avoided by following the simple diagnostic analysis suggested in the CSAG guidelines (previously discussed in this chapter) and ignoring the 'labels'.

The people who use the 'labels' often have very strong and fixed ideas on the treatment and advice that they give, based on a diagnosis that you yourself may doubt. If the treatment you are receiving is not working, question it and if necessary ask for it to be changed. This all goes to show how essential it is that you only consult properly qualified professionals (see the list of relevant organizations, Appendix 3).

5. Neck pain

All the points made in this chapter are as relevant for people suffering from neck pain as for those suffering back pain.

Conclusion

The CSAG guidelines have transformed diagnosis for both the clinician and the patient, simplifying the way neck and pain are classified and therefore handled. For you, they provide a system which is reassuringly easy to understand, allowing you to see for yourself which diagnostic group you fit into, and why.

Key points

1. A specific and accurate diagnosis is at present impossible in most cases of neck and back pain.

2. If you have a 'numb bum' or bladder trouble, with back or leg pain, contact your doctor IMMEDIATELY.

3. If you have a 'red flag' pain (less than one per cent of cases) you will be identified and urgently referred to the appropriate specialist.

4. If you have nerve root pain (less than five per cent of cases) it is highly likely that you will be successfully managed in primary care.

5. For simple neck or back pain (about 95 per cent of cases) there is a 90 per cent recovery rate in six weeks.

6. This straightforward diagnostic system could even allow you to diagnose yourself!

7. It means that the many diagnostic 'labels' that were and still are such a source of confusion and worry can be ignored.

8. The advice and treatment offered by any clinician who still uses the diagnostic 'labels' should be regarded with caution if they are not working.

9. All this information about diagnosis relates as much to neck pain as to back pain.

6

Your experience of acute (short-lived) back and neck pain

Introduction

As we mentioned in the introduction, you will want to know what causes neck and back pain, how it affects you, what the clinicians will do about it, and what you yourself can do about it. In this chapter we discuss what it does to you and what you may think and feel about it.

In February 1994 the National Back Pain Association (NBPA) commissioned research into the experiences of people in the UK with back pain. The research was undertaken by Myradh Kinloch of the Faculty of Human Sciences at Kingston University. We are grateful to her and the NBPA for discussing their findings with us and providing a much clearer, fact-based idea of what is actually happening to you.

Objectives

1. We discuss how you cope with an acute attack NOW, how acute pain disables you, and how quickly you recover.

2. We describe how you think you got your pain, your doctor's diagnosis, and how, at times, you endure more than you should.

3. We consider your current treatment, special investigations, referral, and alternative therapy.

4. We deal with your experience of neck pain.

1. The effects of and recovery from an acute attack

How do you cope with an acute attack?

Just under half of all the people who suffer from an acute attack of back pain or backache cope with it themselves, without consulting anybody at all. This finding, supported by several surveys, is contrary to the commonly held view that people with back or neck pain are not self-reliant.

Your disability in an acute attack

Of those who suffer acute pain around half are unable to use any form of transport during the episode, a third cannot undertake normal household duties, and a third are dependent on another person, for a while, for personal hygiene, dressing, and so on. In other words, a large proportion are severely disabled for a few days during an attack.

In Chapter 7 we suggest that you should not stay in bed for more than three days in an acute attack. In fact, many of you have little choice but to do so!

How quickly do you recover?

A recent paper has shown that 90 per cent of patients with lower back pain stop consulting their doctor within three months despite the fact that 35 per cent of them will still be suffering from the pain and its related disability. There is also a 66 per cent recurrence rate in the first year. (The implications of these statistics for you are discussed in Chapter 16.)

If you suffer a recurrence, you should not consider it unusual but should handle it as an acute attack (see Chapter 8).

2. Causes of pain, the diagnosis, and the need for a consultation

How did you get your pain in the first place?

With regard to what causes your pain, three quarters of you could easily explain why you thought you had symptoms, although the reasons might be very general. About half of you could identify a specific event or events (more often than not associated with leisure activities such as playing sport, dancing, taking exercise, gardening, or doing DIY) which you believe could have triggered off the pain in the first place. Of those who suspect that their problems originate at work, only a minute proportion actually hold their employer responsible. (This is important in view of the widely-held prejudice that back pain is a kind of 'malingerer's charter'.)

Your doctor's diagnosis

Just over half of you are satisfied with this—but obviously that means many of you are not!

Some years ago a doctor was representing the NBPA on a television programme alongside other clinicians such as hospital consultants, osteopaths, and so on. The audience consisted principally of people suffering from chronic back and neck pain. Of all the clinicians, the audience was unanimously critical of doctors—not because they had failed to make them better (because they felt nobody had), but because they had failed to investigate their problem thoroughly enough. On each hospital visit, a proper history and examination had been undertaken; however, during visits to doctors' surgeries, often very little history had been taken and, in most cases, the patient had not even been examined.

This degree of dissatisfaction is unique to this area of medicine and it is unfortunate that the doctor bears the brunt of the blame since he or she is likely to have received little or no training in back and neck problems (despite how common they are). As part of the CSAG guidelines, major educational initiatives are now under way at both undergraduate and postgraduate level.

Unwitting endurance

Nearly a third of those who do consult their doctor have complete confidence in the diagnosis given and do not go back to him or her unless forced to by the need for a sickness certificate or because they have become completely disabled by their pain. The remainder who make up the figure who consult a doctor to nearly 50 per cent, want to discuss the matter further with the doctor, but don't because they are reluctant to bother him or her. Instead, these patients adopt a 'grin and bear it' attitude to their pain. Whilst such stoicism shows courage and consideration, new evidence shows that it increases the risk of the pain becoming chronic (persistent). So, if pain continues for more than a few days, you should see your doctor to get treatment.

3. Your current treatment and alternatives

Treatment by your doctor

Doctors provide three broad types of treatment:

1. Passive: bed rest, traction, collars, and corsets. At present, just over half of patients receive this type of treatment of whom only another half are prescribed medication.
2. Active: referral for physiotherapy, hydrotherapy, and special exercises. About a third of those in the first group additionally receive this treatment.
3. Invasive: referral for spinal injections such as epidurals, manipulation under anaesthesia, and, in a tiny minority of cases, surgery.

As discussed in Chapter 7, the CSAG guidelines suggest radical change with far greater emphasis given to active treatment.

Investigations

Doctors often request investigations, the most usual being a plain X-ray of the spine. Blood tests are sometimes, but less frequently, ordered. Investigations are fully discussed in Chapter 12.

Referral

About half of doctors' referrals are to physio-therapists; most of the other half are to ortho-paedic surgeons. Again, the CSAG guidelines suggest important changes which are described in Chapter 7.

Alternative treatments

Just under half the people who suffer from neck and back pain do consult an alternative practi-tioner such as an osteopath or chiropractor—two-thirds of their own accord, the rest following referral or recommendation. Those who do not seek alternative treatments may be worried that their doctor might be offended or might simply disapprove; perhaps they are not aware of what is available to them. However, the majority of those who see an alternative practitioner are satisfied with the treatment they receive and in fact many judge the alternative therapy to be more effective than conventional treatment (even though it may take longer to work). Of course, most alternative therapy is provided privately, so a practitioner can devote much more time to a consultation than can a NHS doctor. The advice now though is for doctors to involve themselves in the cases in much more detail, or else to suggest referral earlier. (See Chapter 7.)

4. Your experience of neck pain

All the points made in this chapter are as relevant for those suffering from neck pain as from back pain.

Conclusion

With all the new information available on what actually happens to you when you suffer with acute back and neck pain and how you feel about it, there is a compulsion to change the approach to the diagnosis, management, and investigation of your pain. (For example, advice given in a book we published as recently as 1993 is already out of date.) For any changes to be effective, however, it is important that you are aware of them and have a relationship with your clinician that is one of active participation.

Key points

1. Many of you deal with your back and neck pain without any help from anyone.

2. Many people are severely disabled for the first few days of an acute attack.

3. Recent evidence indicates that attacks of back and neck pain do not clear as quickly and completely as had been thought in the past.

4. Most of you are satisfied with your doctor and the treatment given.

5. Just under half of you have tried alternative therapies and find them effective, although they take longer to work than conventional treatments.

6. In the light of new information, the diagnosis, treatment, investigation, and referral offered by doctors should change greatly in the future.

7. For any changes to work well your active involvement and co-operation are vital.

8. All this information relates as much to neck as to back pain.

7
Management of your acute pain

Introduction

In view of the fact that back and neck pain is a growing problem, it would seem that traditional NHS management is not a success and that present methods of treatment do not work. Up until now, little has changed. However, the CSAG guidelines are prompting major initiatives.

Objectives

1. We look at the role of your doctor as defined by the CSAG guidelines.
2. We discuss the new approach to bed rest.
3. We review the new emphasis given to manipulation, exercise, and active rehabilitation.
4. We show why it pays you to stay at work if possible.

5. We explain why you are the key to this policy.
6. We discuss the management of sciatica.
7. We deal with the management of acute neck pain.

1. Your doctor

The guidelines recognize and accept that simple backache should be managed, investigated, and treated mainly in primary care rather than as a specialist problem. As such, the key person in the treatment is your doctor. Armed with accurate, up-to-date information about backache and advice about how to manage it, you can actively participate, with your doctor, in the management of your pain. Hopefully, this will prevent your acute pain becoming chronic. Nevertheless, there is much that can be done for those suffering from chronic neck and back pain, as we shall show in Chapters 10 and 11.

2. Bed rest

Traditionally, bed rest has been regarded as a standard medical treatment for back pain. We now know, however, that there is no advantage in staying in bed for more than three days and that, in general, to stay in bed for longer than you absolutely have to because of the severity of your pain could be potentially harmful for you. The exception to this is for those suffering from nerve root pain (see Chapter 5), for whom a stay in bed of up to two weeks may be advised.

The RCGP has evidence that bed rest can actually make people weaker, unfit, and more prone to depression. Indeed, it can prolong the trouble, rather than treat it. So, the best advice is to stay out of bed if at all possible—even if it hurts.

3. Physical therapy (manipulation), exercise, and active rehabilitation

Physical therapy

The CSAG guidelines point the way to a dramatic change in medical policy with regard to the management of back pain. They state that if the pain lasts for more than a few days, then physical therapists—osteopaths, chiropractors, physiotherapists, and doctors who have been taught to manipulate—should become involved in treatment. Traditionally viewed with suspicion by the medical profession, physical therapy (manipulation) is now regarded as offering an effective and safe form of pain relief for many patients—a view strongly reinforced by scientific work, much of it carried out in the USA. Manipulation is particularly helpful with acute and recurring back or neck pain; it has been shown to be useful, although less so, with chronic and nerve root pain.

There are three key recommendations from the CSAG:

1. Therapists should see any patients selected by doctors within 72 hours.

2. Doctors should routinely refer patients to therapists within two weeks.

3. ALL patients should be seen by therapists within six weeks.

The essential point is that that your doctor should be willing to refer you to a physical therapist—and to refer you sooner than in the past. If he or she is not happy to do so, then you should consider taking yourself to such a person, provided always that they are properly qualified and trained and so present no risk to you (see Appendix 3).

Finally, if you are one of the many (about 50 per cent) who don't bother to see a doctor, there is clear evidence that if your pain lasts for more than, say, three days, then you should. Active and early intervention is now known to be effective and can reduce the risk of your problem becoming chronic.

Active rehabilitation and exercise

However, it must be emphasized that manipulation alone is not enough. Therapists should not only aim to relieve pain, but should also work towards the rehabilitation of the patient and the education and involvement of the patient in the management of their pain.

Presently, 55 per cent of treatment that you get from your doctor is passive (pain killers and bed rest) and around a third is active (the addition of other treatments such as hydrotherapy, active exercises, and physiotherapy). These proportions are set to change, however, as it is now known that for a successful final outcome management should also be directed to exercise and activity.

Exercise

There is, as yet, no evidence to suggest that any one particular exercise is better than any other. We know, however, that walking, cycling and swimming are effective not only in improving flexibility but also in reducing pain. Exercise should be started as soon as possible—certainly within the first two weeks—and gradually increased.

Activity

An active rehabilitation programme uses exercises but its main emphasis is on restoring full function and regaining physical fitness. It concentrates on progressively increased quotas of activity rather than on symptoms of pain. In fact, an increase in pain when exercise or activity is begun is common. There is a crucial difference between 'hurt' and 'harm'. It is natural to assume that pain is a warning to stop doing whatever brings it on. With regard to back and neck pain, however, it will not cause any new harm or damage unless it is very severe. Indeed, by not persisting with the exercise, you run the risk of the problem becoming chronic. (So, previous advice to patients, given by many clinicians, to stop if it hurts, is now obsolete!)

Early activity is strongly encouraged since:

1. it is not harmful;
2. it reduces pain in the long run;
3. physical fitness is beneficial.

Other treatments

Other treatments include injections (for example, facet, epidural, trigger point) and some physical treatments (heat and cold, acupuncture, TENS, and so on). All these, and many others, are discussed in Chapter 9.

4. Stay at work

Previously, patients have often asked for certificates to stay off work, and doctors have readily given them, because both believed it was the right thing to do. This may have unwittingly caused more harm since we now know that patients treated with active exercise and an early return to work have fewer recurrences of problems, less additional time off, and less health care over the next two years. You should be advised to give up work only if there is a likelihood that you will come to harm if you continue.

5. You are the key

The changes outlined in this chapter involve you in a much closer partnership with your doctor or physical therapist, in the management of your pain, than in the past. In order for the policy to work you will need more information from your doctor or physical therapist and advice on how to handle the situation. Up-to-date, well-designed educational material, suitable for both the patient and the general public, is required.

The three key areas in which you need information are:

1. expectations about rapid recovery; awareness of the possible recurrence of symptoms (most patients have some recurrence of back and neck pain and, as long as you are aware of this fact, you are less likely to be distressed if it happens to you);

2. safe and proven methods of symptom control (see Chapters 12 and 13);

3. safe and reasonable activity (remembering to keep active, to exercise, and to stay at work if you possibly can).

6. The management of sciatica

Sciatica (pain in the leg) may be due to nerve root problems. Management of its pain is essentially the same as for simple back pain, with a few differences—more painkillers may be needed initially; bed rest may be required for up to two weeks (but more should be avoided); and progress is likely to be slower.

7. Management of neck pain

All the points made in this chapter relate as much to neck pain as to back pain.

Conclusion

A complete change of management policy, based on the latest scientific evidence, has taken place.

The new approach gives you a key role to play, sharing responsibility for your recovery with your doctor or therapist. Central to the success of the policy is the need for you to be fully informed.

Key points

1. The doctor or therapist is crucial in the new management policy.
2. Bed rest for more than three days should be avoided in cases of simple neck and back pain.
3. Manipulation is a key therapy.
4. Exercise and physical activity relieves pain and speeds recovery.
5. Loss of work should be avoided if at all possible.
6. The management of sciatica is essentially the same, but may require a longer recovery period.
7. Your personal participation and responsibility in management and rehabilitation is essential.
8. All this advice applies equally to people suffering with neck pain as to those with back pain.

8
Self-help—what you can do about your acute pain

Introduction

The last chapter outlined new advice for the management of acute back and neck pain—namely, stay out of bed, consider manipulation, exercise, stay active, and continue working. In this chapter we spell out the practicalities of this advice as it is applied on 'day one', 'day four', and 'day seven and beyond'.

Objectives

1. For 'day one' we review what you do about your doctor, pain relief, bed rest, heat and cold, manipulation, exercise, activity, and work.

2. We do the same for 'day four'.

3. We repeat this process for 'day seven and beyond'.

4. We discuss specific advice given for treating neck pain (pillows, collars, and exercises).

1. Day one

Being suddenly smitten with acute back or neck pain can be a very frightening experience. However, there is no need to panic—frequently the pain resolves of its own accord and often there is quite rapid improvement.

Your doctor

Do not send for your doctor at this stage as there is little that he or she could do. There are two exceptions to this advice. The first important one is if you develop any problems with your bladder or bowels, a 'numb bum', or pins and needles and weakness in both legs. Should this happen contact your doctor right away as these serious (though extremely rare) symptoms may indicate a need for surgery. The second reason for contacting your doctor on day one is if the pain is excruciating. If this is the case he or she may refer you for urgent physical therapy or to a pain clinic for immediate pain relief.

Bed rest

The best advice is not to go to bed at all. However, for about a third of you the pain will be so severe at the onset that you will be immobilized. Take comfort though from the fact that most people in this situation improve greatly within three days.

There are a number of useful tips for those of you forced to take to your bed. Firstly, there is much debate on the best kind of bed for bad backs. The simple answer is that the best bed for you is the one in which you are most comfortable, be it hard or soft. If you think your bed is too hard, then it is worth trying to find a softer one. On the other hand, if it seems too soft, you can either put a board under the mattress (which may or may not help) or put the mattress on the floor. Certainly do not buy a special 'orthopaedic' bed or any other item without trying it out first. Anyway, such a purchase may well be unnecessary in an acute attack because of the high likelihood of the problem resolving itself. (For those of you with chronic pain, we discuss this issue further in Chapter 11.)

It is difficult to eat and drink in bed; you may find it helps to use a bent straw for drinking. It is sensible to eat or drink as little as possible in the early stages, so as to reduce the need to go to the toilet. Do not worry if you are slightly constipated for this is quite normal in anyone confined to bed. When you do have to go, try to get to the bathroom; perching on a bedpan can be problematic. To get out of bed when you are in pain, it is best to roll to the edge of the bed, bring your knees up, and drop your feet over the side. Then sit up sideways and use a chair near the bed for support. You may find it more comfortable to crawl than to try and walk.

Pain relief

Painkillers can be very helpful in the first two or three days, not only in making you feel more comfortable but also, by relieving pain, in allowing you to do necessary exercise and activity. Paracetamol, aspirin, or an anti-inflammatory drug such as Nurofen can be used, but the last two have potential side-effects and certainly should not be taken if you have suffered from ulcers. You may well have a preference for a particular painkiller that has worked on other occasions—try that first. The advice now is to take regular doses of, say, two tablets every four or six hours, rather than on an 'as and when' basis. (The management of chronic pain requires a different approach which is detailed later in the book.)

A hot water bottle applied to the part that hurts most is often helpful, but remember that you need to keep it there for at least 20 minutes to get the full advantage. If it is too hot on its own, wrap it in a towel. Some people find an ice-pack more beneficial. A packet of frozen peas makes a satisfactory home-made ice-pack; it will mould itself to your shape and you can return it to the freezer after use. If heat does not work, try cold, and vice versa. Some find it most helpful to alternate, perhaps several times, between heat and cold.

Ointments, such as Algipan, can be helpful and are harmless. Applying the ointment involves gentle massage, which may bring comfort in itself—although you must tell whoever is doing the massage to stop if it hurts you.

Manipulation

As discussed in the previous chapter, this is not indicated at this stage unless your doctor feels that the severity of your pain justifies it.

Exercise

You may well be immobilized by the severity of your pain, making any exercise impossible to begin with. On the other hand, you should try to get moving as soon as you can; the painkillers will enable you to start exercise and activity without delay. At the moment there is no evidence to recommend one particular exercise above another, although walking, swimming, and cycling are all to be encouraged. You can organize your own exercise programme—begin with a small amount and gradually do more and more each day. Remember, as we have already explained, 'hurt' does not mean 'harm' and there are definite advantages to be gained by putting up with a certain amount of pain initially.

Activity

The same advice applies to activity—start as soon as you can and build back to normal as quickly as you can. As with exercise, plan your own programme, breaking up your day with different jobs and activities so that you are neither sitting nor lying for long periods. Gradually increase what you do, day by day.

The workplace

Obviously, if you are unable to move, you have to go to bed. But if you possibly can, stay at work despite the pain. If you explain to your boss and/or colleagues what is happening, they may well help out with some of your work, or your boss may put you on light duties for a time.

2. Day four

Your doctor

Day four is something of a watershed because this is the time you should be alerting your doctor if you are not improving or still have a lot of pain. His or her first priority will be to ensure that you do not have a 'red flag' pain but simple back or neck pain or a nerve root problem.

Bed rest

Both you and your doctor should be concerned if, at this point, you are still in bed, since we now know that after three days bed rest is harmful. Most patients will be out of bed; if you are not, particular effort should be made.

Painkillers

The advice on painkillers is exactly as for day one, and for the same reasons—they help to get you out of bed and engaging in exercise and activity.

Manipulation

Because of the time that has now elapsed both you and your doctor should be giving this serious consideration; it is now indicated.

Exercise and activity

These are now of increasing importance, and you should make every effort to do more and more.

The workplace

Again, make every effort to stay at or go back to work.

3. Day seven and beyond

Your doctor

If your doctor has not already treated you with physical therapy, he or she should be referring you to a therapist. Patients with simple back and neck pain (95 per cent) should have had physical therapy routinely within two weeks; all patients should have seen a therapist within six. If your doctor will not refer you, then consider making your own arrangements to see a therapist.

Painkillers

The same advice as for day one and day four, and for the same reasons.

Manipulation

See the advice given under 'your doctor' .

Exercise, activity, and the workplace

The same advice as before still applies, but is now of increasing urgency.

4. Specific advice for neck pain

All the advice in this chapter applies as much to neck pain as it does to back pain, and should be followed just as seriously and for exactly the same reasons. On the other hand, there are a few problems that affect specifically those suffering with neck pain.

Collars

Although at present there is no hard evidence about the value or otherwise of collars, many of those suffering with acute neck pain do find them beneficial. It is very easy to make yourself a collar from just a newspaper. Fold it to make a strip about four inches wide and about eighteen inches to two feet long and wrap it around your neck like a scarf, adjusting it so that it is neither too loose nor too painful. Secure it with adhesive tape. In the same way you can also make a collar from latex rubber sponge. Time spent moulding and trimming the latex rubber sponge collar is well worthwhile. The guiding principle is that if a collar makes you feel more comfortable, then wear one; if it doesn't, then don't.

Pillows

These can be of a great help to those suffering with neck pain and you should experiment to discover whether one, two, or no pillows suits you best. You might well try out a 'butterfly' pillow. This is a pillow with the contents shaken out to either end, the centre being placed at the nape of the neck. This will often provide relief.

Exercise

Although there is no proof of which specific exercises are best, if you find one that helps you, and it does not increase the pain, then do it. It can do no harm.

Conclusion

Nowadays, you have as important a role to play as any clinician. Their job is to exclude the 'red flags' and to arrange for or give you physical therapy at the appropriate time. Whilst this treatment is often very effective in relieving the pain, it must be combined with aggressive exercise and activity which is started as soon as possible and is under your control, pushed to the limits of your discomfort. Your clinician can help you plan the exercise and activity, but only you know the limits of your discomfort, and therefore the burden of how far and how fast to go lies with you. You should involve your family and your work colleagues if necessary.

Current advice to continue ordinary activity can relieve symptoms of an acute attack as well as, or even quicker than, traditional treatment with painkillers and bed rest. It will also result in less chronic disability and less time off work. As new information emerges, and reviews of these guidelines may become necessary, it is essential that you keep up to date with the current position.

Key points

1. Start to work on the problem as soon as possible.

2. Do as much exercise and activity as you can.

3. If needed, take painkillers regularly and in full doses—they will help you to get on with your 'programme' of exercise and activity.

4. Involve your clinician from day four, but not before—unless your pain is very severe or you develop a 'numb bum' or bowel or bladder problems.

5. If your clinician does not agree to referral for physical therapy, organize it for yourself, making sure you choose a fully qualified therapist.

6. Involve your family and work colleagues if necessary.

7. All this advice is equally applicable for neck pain as for back pain.

9

Your experience of chronic (persistent) back and neck pain

Introduction

Acute (short-lived) and chronic (persistent) pain produce very different problems. A 'chronic pain state' refers to chronic pain from any cause and presents with certain generic symptoms and problems, as applicable to chronic back and neck pain as to any other chronic pain.

One key difference between acute and chronic pain is that the latter inevitably has psychological consequences that have to be taken account of by your doctor and, if the situation is to be handled properly, by you. We now have a much clearer picture about the many ways in which chronic back and neck pain intrude into your life, enabling us to give more precise advice to you and the clinicians on how to handle the situation.

Objectives

1. We look at your feelings about and understanding of your pain, and whether it is 'all in the mind'.

2. We discuss how pain can affect you at work, cost you money, and alter your activities (including leisure pursuits).

3. We describe how you react to these difficulties and how your disability may be even greater than you realize.

4. We explain how you can tackle all this and the importance of not becoming a back pain 'reject'.

5. We review the situation specifically in relation to chronic neck pain.

1. The psychological consequences

The psychologist uses the term 'affect' to describe the way you feel about pain. As the pain persists, you are likely to become depressed, frightened, and irritable. These changes will inevitably affect those around you such as your family, friends, employer, and colleagues. The longer the pain lasts, the greater the risk that you will become seriously depressed; 10 per cent of pain clinic patients have a treatable depressive illness. So if you feel it is getting you down, don't be afraid of seeking help from your doctor—remember, everybody in this situation is affected to some degree.

The psychologists call the way you understand your pain, 'cognition'. Your understanding will play a big part in what you think and feel about your situation. For example, if you believe that your neck pain is caused by a serious disease, you will be much more worried than if you have been reassured that that is not the case. As we have stressed so many times, it is therefore vital that you have adequate and reliable information about your condition, and can 'talk it through' with someone. Unfortunately, at the moment this does not happen enough.

Pain behaviour is what you actually DO because of your pain—for example, how many tablets you take; how much time you spend in bed; how your pain affects your ability to do jobs both at home and work; and how you get on with those around you. Chapter 10 describes how, if your condition is to improve as much as it can, elements of pain behaviour can be identified and then removed.

So, both physical and psychological factors (mind and body) interact to produce the experience we call pain. To make the point even more forcibly, if you have had pain for six weeks it is now strongly recommended that you have a 'biopsychosocial' assessment (see Chapter 10)—a check-up that includes routinely some psychological assessment. This leads to another significant point. Many patients and, alas, some doctors, believe that the pain is 'all in the mind'. There is, however, no evidence to support this opinion.

2. Work, money, and activities

Work worries

It is natural that being off work is a major concern for all involved; it is one of the most common queries for the NBPA helpline (see Chapter 16). Those people who work part-time (the majority of whom are women) feel particularly anxious at the possibility of losing their jobs because they fear there may be little chance of getting other work. As a result, they may often struggle through their work, frequently to spend the following day or days in bed because of the pain. This in turn places a burden on their families. Thus your pain can affect every aspect of your life.

Finance

Around a third of you with chronic pain will spend money because of it, for example, buying furniture or equipment as a means of self-help, altering living spaces, or moving fixtures and fittings.

Activities

Nearly a third of you stop using upstairs rooms or working in the garden; another third cut down gardening to essential duties.

Your pain may well have a devastating effect on your social life, as other common activities become severely restricted—around a quarter of patients stop visiting pubs, clubs, or friends; a similar proportion of you give up your normal means of exercise (which often means that you take no exercise at all); and yet another quarter give up hobbies such as DIY. This can lead to a feeling of isolation.

3. Your personal disability

Many of you would probably not recognize, or want to admit, that you have a disability, and would claim to be able to perform all your tasks normally, all of the time. But in fact, disability is not only very common but is also a greater problem than many of you realize: you will show signs of change. For example, you may do things slowly or 'in your own time'; perhaps you take taxis, when once you would have walked. This is particularly noticeable in the elderly. Phrases commonly used to disguise the level of disability include ' I don't need as much as I used to' (when referring to shopping) and 'I don't go out much these days' (when referring to taking walks).

4. How can you tackle the problem?

As described, persistent pain is not only bad enough in itself but can have many crippling effects on you. You may not even realize what is happening, which is why, in this chapter, we have given you a profile of how chronic pain manifests itself. We will show you how you can help yourself, in Chapter 11, and the great help others can give you, in Chapter 10.

Chronic back and neck pain is much more than a baffling, depressing, and miserable existence. It is very easy to passively accept that nothing more can be done about it—that it is natural 'wear and tear'. Nothing could be further from the truth! Certainly the problems are complex and very personal (even more so than for acute pain), but with thought and understanding, and if you are fully informed and involved, they can be identified and tackled.

The main thing is to realize that the more you do, the less disabled you are. Do not become a back or neck pain 'reject'. Remember that 'hurt' is not the same as 'harm' (see Chapter 7) and to obtain normal function (or as near it as you can) it is worth putting up with some pain. Maybe you cannot beat your pain, but you can go a very long way to stop it beating you and your family.

5. Your experience of neck pain

The profile given in this chapter is as relevant for those suffering chronic neck pain, as back pain.

Conclusion

Because the effects of chronic back and neck pain are so many and so complicated, it can be difficult to find the best solution. On the other hand, as we show in Chapter 10, a good outcome can be achieved in most cases. Nowadays there is much that can and is being done; there has never been a time when it made less sense for you to 'give up'.

Key points

1. Chronic pain invariably has psychological consequences.

2. There is no evidence with back and neck pain that it is 'all in the mind'.

3. Chronic pain can involve not only work loss but also intrudes into almost every aspect of your life.

4. Disability affects more than half of those suffering from back and neck pain—and probably many more.

5. If this level of disability is understood, you can do much to help overcome it.

6. The outcome can be very good indeed.

7. All this is as true for neck pain as back pain.

10
Management of your chronic pain

Introduction

As with acute pain, the present system for managing chronic pain does not work as well as it should. The CSAG guidelines propose major changes.

Objectives

1. We describe the present hospital referral system and show why a multidisciplinary back and neck pain rehabilitation service and bio-psychosocial assessment (as recommended in the guidelines) are necessary.

2. We explain why the acknowledgement of your pain is important and that the main aim is not pain relief but a reduction in the level of your disability so that you can function normally (or as near normally as possible).

3. We look at exercise, the pain psychologist (and how he or she helps you take control of your

life), and the essential part played by your family.

4. We assess the attempts to reduce the disability caused by your pain.

5. We review the importance of your role in this.

6. We deal with the specifics of neck pain.

1. The present situation and suggestions for change

At the moment, there are not enough hospital specialists, including many of the consultants working in rheumatology and orthopaedic surgery, with a particular interest in back and neck pain. Having been referred to a specialist, you may well be told that you do not have an inflammatory disease or need an operation and will be sent back to your doctor with nothing having been done. Unfortunately, this all takes quite a lot of time and in the meanwhile your problem is more likely to become chronic—a situation which obviously should be avoided if possible.

A multidisciplinary back and neck pain rehabilitation service

As described in Chapter 9, chronic pain is a complicated condition; as such it requires a complex response. No single specialist is likely to be as helpful as a group of people who together have all the necessary skills and experience to handle the problems. Such a multidisciplinary service is already well established at the larger pain clinics, where back pain currently constitutes between 25 and 50 per cent of the referrals they receive. Unfortunately, at the moment, many pain clinics are small and only provide services for altering medication and giving injections. This is not enough to sort out the problem of chronic pain in all its complexity.

The CSAG guidelines recommend more pain clinics, staffed by teams comprising physiotherapists, psychologists, sometimes occupational therapists, and nurses experienced in pain management. Such multidisciplinary teams:

1. stress that traditional medical management is not enough;

2. urge you to do more and more for yourself, offering advice on how this is possible;

3. identify and eliminate your pain behaviour, restoring you to normal physical condition (or as near as possible) with a graduated programme of exercise, and activity.

Any back pain rehabilitation service will have very different aims, resources, and referral patterns to those services for the management of patients with 'red flag' conditions (for example, serious spinal pathology or multiple nerve root pain). It will be a service for patients who have failed to recover from 'mechanical' problems.

The biopsychosocial assessment (or six-week check-up)

It is clear that chronic disability has associated psychological and social problems which may develop because of the pain itself or because treatment has failed. For whatever reason they develop, these problems can become as important, or even more important, than the original pain itself. A biopsychosocial assessment looks at all these aspects of your pain. The guidelines recommend that if you still have back and neck pain after six weeks you should have such an assessment.

2. Is your pain real?

Many patients question whether their pain is real and worthy of consideration. The first, and most valuable thing, that a pain clinic doctor must do is to assure you that you are believed and that your pain is genuine. Chapter 11 looks at how serious an issue this is for you.

The aims of the pain clinic

It is very characteristic of people with chronic pain who are attending a pain clinic that, despite many failed attempts to relieve their pain, they are still hoping for complete pain relief. (One major pain clinic excludes people who are looking for a 'cure'.) Some may say that they are not looking for a total 'cure', but secretly still hope for such. The value of these clinics is that they educate the patients into having priorities other than getting rid of the pain. They tackle the problems that develop in patients with chronic sickness, which include an overdependence on doctors, a need to find a medical solution for their condition, and a tendency to want others to take control of their lives. By the end of their pain clinic programme, patients may admit that although their pain is the same, they have learnt much that can change their lives.

Of course it is only natural that people should hope to have their pain relieved, and pain clinics do have their successes—they relieve pain for about 30 to 40 per cent of patients, and reduce it for another 20 per cent. But their principal function is to reduce the level of disability you suffer because of your back and neck pain.

3. Improving the quality of your life

The importance of exercise

Exercise and activity are just as important in the management of chronic pain as of acute pain. They produce good results in patients—not necessarily by directly reducing pain—but by increasing movement, muscle strength, and mobility.

The pain psychologist

The pain psychologist is a key member of the team at the pain clinic or rehabilitation service, working, not to eliminate your chronic pain, but to reduce or abolish the disability that it brings with it. Their approach may or may not lessen the frequency or intensity of your pain, but it should increase your activities and thereby improve the quality of your life.

First, the psychologist explores your understanding of your problem, in order to identify and correct any misconceptions. Then, you are taught about the way you think about your pain (cognition), the way you feel about it (affect), and how you behave (the things you do in response to it). These three factors influence each other in a way that can make your problems persist or even get worse. If you are aware of how they interact all the time, you can work to positively improve the situation.

You may resent being seen by a psychologist, believing that people will therefore think that you are mad or malingering. However, as chronic pain has undeniable psychological elements, the psychologist can do much to help you.

Case history: a reluctant success

We wanted to refer one of our patients, a middle-aged woman with chronic neck pain, to a pain clinic. Being a cautious person she enquired closely as to what this would involve. She was not pleased to learn that she would be seen by a psychologist, believing that this meant that we obviously thought that she was either faking her pain or that she was mad. Nothing we said placated her and she refused her referral point-blank. As it happened, a neighbour went to the local clinic and was very happy with the outcome. Our patient subsequently returned to us and said that she was prepared to try. She was pleasantly surprised at how successful it was—although remaining wary!

Taking control of your life

Clinicians at the pain clinic or back pain service

will encourage you to plan your own life and to take charge of your situation. Many treatments require you to keep a diary, so that you may understand what is happening to you. You then set yourself realistic levels of activity which are not too high (since if you fail due to your pain, you will be more depressed and inclined to give up) and which can be progressively increased each day.

There is much evidence that the more pain-killers you take, the worse off you become. So, one of the first things most pain clinics will aim to do is to cut down on your use of these drugs.

Bed rest can also easily become a pain behaviour. So, you will be urged to cut this down gradually and, instead, to take a more positive attitude to your condition. For example, we now know that the more exercise you take, the less likely you are to complain about your pain; you are distracted by what you are actually doing, rather than brooding over your situation.

At the pain clinic you are also taught the skills of relaxation and controlled breathing. These and other similar techniques, by giving you something you can do yourself to control your pain, make you feel less helpless. This is not only useful but also boosts your morale—and morale is a key factor for anyone suffering from chronic pain. If you feel miserable, you are NOT being feeble; misery is a understandable reaction to pain.

Using everything taught at the pain clinic will give you an understanding of your problem and a range of responses and practical hints to help you to regain control of your life. You can do more and live a fuller and more active life.

Your family

Your family may feel as helpless, as ignorant, and, at times, as desperate as you. They may not understand your problem; they may feel defeated by it and not know how they can help you. But families are welcome at pain clinics and, when given the explanations that you are given, will understand the aims of your treatment and the part they can play.

Usually the pain clinic will insist on your family being involved in the treatment programme, since they can prompt you to achieve your goals by encouraging you and preventing you from slipping back into bad habits. You and your family are considered as a single unit, working together towards your recovery.

4. How successful are these teams?

You may question how successful these pain management teams are, given that the relief of pain is only achieved in about half the patients. But in fact most teams produce reductions in invalid behaviour, drug consumption, and demand for medical and social services in around 85 per cent of the patients they see. There is obviously much they can do.

5. What is your role?

It is important that you know what is happening to you and your family, and why. The pain clinic programmes give you an understanding of your problem and advice as to how to improve your everyday life, but the person who has the most control over the situation is you. Central to the matter is your realization that you are not helpless, defeated, and rejected and that, with the right help and the right attitude, you can do much for yourself. You have to identify and eliminate those factors that are harmful and concentrate on those that give positive results.

5. Management of neck pain

All the points made in this chapter relate as much to the management of chronic neck pain as to chronic back pain.

Conclusion

Everybody admits that chronic pain is more difficult to manage than acute pain. It is excellent therefore that a multidisciplinary team can effect change in 85 per cent of patients. The aim is to provide a specific, local back and neck pain service nationwide. Obviously this will take time, but there is now evidence that these services are beginning to be set up. Whilst this is going on, the essentially common sense principles that they operate on can be formally recommended to and acted on by doctors and physical therapists. They can likewise be acted on by you.

Key points

1. Because your chronic pain problems are complex they are best handled by a multi-disciplinary team.

2. Pain relief is not the primary aim—although good results are achieved in this respect.

3. The main aim is the reduction of your disability for which there is an excellent 85 per cent success rate.

4, The principles used are basically common sense and can be followed by you at home or in your workplace.

5. If you need information and personal involvement in handling acute pain, you require both all the more in dealing with your chronic pain.

6. All this advice applies equally to people suffering with neck pain as to those with back pain.

11

Self-help—what you can do about your chronic pain

Introduction

In Chapter 8 we showed how crucial self-help is in the management of acute back and neck pain. Many believe it to be, together with manipulation, the main way to prevent loss of work and chronic pain. In the last chapter we demonstrated how pain clinics manage, basically by programmes of increasing exercise and activity, to often relieve chronic pain and, much more significantly, to reduce the level of disability caused by it. Thus, the same methods are used nowadays in the management of both acute and chronic pain—and for the same reasons (less time off work, less pain, and less disability).

Before progress can be made, firstly, your pain has to be accepted as genuine by all concerned and, secondly, you need to acknowledge how much your pain is disabling you. Many people are surprised, when they go through their plan of daily activities, to discover how disabled they have become. Many fail to do more not because it hurts, but because it might. An extreme example of this is a woman who had not shopped for two years because she feared that it might provoke her neck pain that had, in fact, cleared up 18 months before. She was persuaded to try a cautious amount of shopping and to increasingly do more and more. She was fine.

Patients basically divide into two types—the 'avoiders' and the 'copers'. To avoid pain or the risk of it, through not doing things, makes nothing better and may in fact make things worse. By doing everything that you can, despite some pain, you are coping. Chapter 7 included convincing evidence that being a 'coper' brings significant benefits. A positive attitude on your part is crucial, combined with a sensible approach of 'start small', do not overdo it, and build up gradually.

The essential point, as with self-help for acute pain, is that 'hurt' does not necessarily imply 'harm'. To put up with a certain amount of pain is worth it to avoid having your life unnecessarily dominated by it. This is the more so when you realize that exercise and activity can actually help to relieve pain.

Results achieved by pain clinics can be good provided that the goals are clearly stated and, above all, are realistic. Patients need to be aware that the aim is not to cure their pain (although it may well be diminished) but rather, with their help and co-operation, to enable them to lead a more active and normal life. Everybody would, of course, rather be completely free from pain. Nevertheless, many are often pleased and grateful for the improvements that are brought about.

This chapter offers advice on how to tackle many activities. However, because everybody's problems are different, there is no one right way to do things. What you personally will find helpful is a matter of trial and error. Increase your activities if you possibly can; giving up is the worst thing that you can do.

Objectives

1. We discuss problems in the home (for example, hoovering, washing the floor, hanging curtains, hanging out washing, ironing, shopping, using the sink and other kitchen working surfaces, cleaning the bath, sitting, shaving, washing your face, applying make-up, making beds, sex, decorating, moving furniture), in the garage, and in the garden.

2. We review problems at work in the office, in heavy industry, and on the assembly line, and for farm workers, construction workers, and lorry drivers.

3. We consider travel—public transport, cars, air travel, cycling, and walking.

4. We list eight golden rules for lifting.

5. We detail the problems for those suffering from neck pain, giving advice on collars, pillows, posture, and activities.

1. Domestic chores

Hoovering

This can cause back and neck problems because you often have to stoop a little, and are pulling or pushing a heavy vibrating machine—all of which puts pressure on your spine. You can reduce the effects by choosing a machine which allows you to stand up straight; this means either one with a long enough handle or one with a flexible suction hose. Whilst you will still be doing as much pulling and pushing, it will be at a more suitable height. Also, you will only have to move the machine itself from time to time.

If you still get pain do the job in several short stints or, if you can afford it, get help with your housework. (The same applies to every household job that causes you back or neck pain and which you have to do or can avoid.)

Washing the floor

It is best to remain standing when cleaning the floor, so you need a long-handled mop or squeegee. You can also avoid putting a strain on your back by doing the cleaning on your hands and knees, provided you keep your back hollowed by sticking your bottom out—advice which goes for many activities which risk causing back pain. It may not be very elegant but it can prevent a great deal of damage. Remember also that it is better to carry two half buckets of water than one full one.

Hanging or removing curtains (or cleaning windows)

Dealing with curtains often puts a strain on your neck and upper back as you are in an awkward position for some time and reaching up to take what may be a considerable weight. There are two things that may help. The first is to stand on something, so that you are working at a more comfortable level—but make sure that what you are standing on is safe! The second is to do the job in several goes—hang or take down one pair of curtains, then do something else for a while before returning for another session.

Hanging out the washing

This presents just the same problems as hanging curtains, maybe made worse by the weight of water in the wet clothes. So either stand on something of a suitable height or bring the line down to the most comfortable level. If hanging out the washing is a frequent activity, it is worth persisting until you have a system that is right for you. Perhaps an adjustable-height drying rack is the answer, if you have the room for it.

Ironing

Frequently you stoop over too low an ironing-board for too long at a time. If you choose to do the ironing sitting down, you obviously need the board quite low, but if you iron standing up you must have the board high enough so that you stand up straight. Whichever position you adopt you will find it less of a strain on your back and neck if the board is at about the level of your navel.

Shopping

You should carry your shopping equally divided between your two hands. You may find a light-weight trolley helpful. Be careful about loading and unloading the car boot with heavy shopping. When doing this keep your back straight and lift from the knees; try not to twist your body as you lift or put down the bags.

At the sink

Long periods may be spent standing in one position at the kitchen sink when preparing vegetables, washing-up, and so on. Unfortunately, most kitchen designers forget that the working height of a sink is its base, which means that you are stooping for much of the time you spend at the sink. Also, most sinks are set some distance from the front edge of the working surface and, as there is seldom enough room to get your feet well under the sink, you have to lean forwards all the time. If you have a back or neck problem you need to consider all these points. If you cannot change the design of your kitchen at least try to avoid working at your sink for any long period of time or do the washing-up in a bowl on the draining-board.

Other kitchen working surfaces

Ideally these should be as near your waist level as possible and you should be able to get your feet close enough to or under the working surface to let your stomach rest against its edge. It is a mistake to plan a kitchen with all the work surfaces at the same height as different tasks and people of different heights necessitate surfaces at different heights. You can vary the height of the surfaces by using different widths of plinth at the base of the units.

High shelves and cupboards present the same problems as curtains and should be dealt with in the same way. And, of course, the height of your oven should not make you stoop or reach.

Sitting in comfort

The easy chair and the sofa are often too soft to give your back the support it needs, or are too low to get in and out of in safety and comfort or to provide the right support to your neck. If you get pain sitting in a soft, low chair, a sensible alternative is a hard, high-backed chair that gives good support. Try not to sit with a rounded back as this may lead to symptoms of back and neck pain.

When watching television, place your chair directly in front of the set. Reading, knitting, or sewing for long periods may give you a neck problem, so do something else if it starts to hurt—do not carry on regardless.

If you do a lot of reading it may help to use a bookstand. However, before buying one (or also one of the many special chairs designed for those who suffer from back pain), borrow one if you can to find out whether or not it helps you. The NBPA has a list of shops that supply this specialist equipment. If you cannot find a chair which supports your back, a lumbar roll or a rolling pin placed in the small of your back may help.

These notes on sitting at home also apply to sitting at work.

Shaving, washing your face, or putting on make-up

Surprisingly all three of these everyday activities are often the cause of back and neck pain—sometimes severe. One reason, of course, may be that you are stooping over the basin for quite a long time. So, think about your position—basically, the straighter, the safer. You may also need to put your mirror higher on the wall or move it so that you do not have to twist to look into it.

Cleaning the bath

This can cause pain when stooping or reaching. Try kneeling or squatting in the bath so that everything is in easy reach; kneeling on the floor beside the bath does not prevent you having to stretch to clean the other side. Incidentally, handholds on the bath are a help for getting in and out of the bath.

Obviously, a shower unit is less problematic for using and cleaning than a bath.

Making the bed

This always involves stooping and reaching and both may be painful. You can reduce the risk by kneeling down when making the bed. You may also find the use of a duvet a great help, as it means you do not have to lift and tuck in bedclothes. Perhaps a higher bed would make life easier for you, both in bedmaking and getting in and out of bed.

The bed is probably the most important piece of furniture in your house; you are likely to spend about 25 years of your life in it. No one bed can be recommended as the best for your back, since every person is different and there are so many possible causes of back pain. The only way to find out which bed is best for you is by trial and error. It is not enough just to lie down on one in a shop; you must try lying in different positions, preferably over a month or so. The NBPA have a list of shops that supply furniture on approval.

When away from home you may find sleeping in a strange bed painful. If you are normally most comfortable on a firm bed, you could take a portable bedboard with you when travelling.

Sex

You may have to ask your partner to adopt unusual positions to accommodate your back or neck problem. The key to a happy sex life is to experiment with different positions until you find one that is comfortable for both of you. If your pain is causing real problems in your sex life, and this is making you or your partner miserable, you should ask for advice from whoever is managing your condition. The NBPA also has a book on sex and back pain that you may find helpful.

Decorating

Skirtings and ceilings are particularly problematic. Skirtings may be best dealt with on your hands and knees with your back hollowed; long-handled rollers may help with ceilings. Working too hard and for too long at one go, with your head in an awkward position, is a recipe for disaster. It is better to split the job into smaller stages. Best of all would be to get someone to do it for you, if you can afford this solution.

Moving furniture

This is best left to other people, but if you have to move furniture, empty cupboards and remove drawers before moving the 'carcass'. A length of strong material, such as upholsterer's webbing, is useful as a sling placed under the piece to be moved and across your shoulders. Allow ample time for moving heavy furniture.

In the garage

Inspecting your car engine means that you will probably spend a long time stooping and reaching. Remember to change your activity as soon as you feel discomfort. If you have a back or neck problem already, take particular care when getting underneath the car and then standing up again.

In the garden

Jobs in the garden are often physically demanding. Some involve stooping and lifting, which may be a cause of painful episodes, and some may need machinery which could be heavy and awkward to use. If you can afford it, it might be best to hire a gardener to do your heavy work; otherwise, follow the advice now given.

Digging

If digging hurts, you can try to reduce the pain by using a spade with a long handle (keeping your back hollow and your bottom sticking out); a larger handle gives you greater leverage. You might also try one of the special spades available through gardening catalogues, which are said to be easier to use. You must train yourself to take a smaller amount of soil on each spadeful and, as with any heavy work in the garden or elsewhere, not to work continuously but to take planned breaks. The same advice applies to using a garden fork.

Hoeing

When using a long-handled hoe, whether a chopping or a pushing type, it may help to keep your back hollowed. However, it is more important to change jobs frequently. With a short-handled hoe, you might consider kneeling down.

Weeding

As far as your back is concerned, weeding is a similar activity to short-handled hoeing. A cushioned mat may be a comfort, but the most important thing is not to do too much for too long.

Mowing the lawn

The dangers here are in stooping to start the machine, manoeuvring a heavy mower around corners, disposing of the cut grass, and the basic height of the lawnmower handles. You may need to change the length of the starting cord, so that you can pull it from handle height instead of having to bend down. Choose the lightest machine you can; electric ones are usually lighter and do not need starting. You may find a hover mower the best.

Even if it seems very small for your lawn, it is better to make more runs with a small machine than to give yourself back or neck pain by using a larger model. Handles vary in height, and if they are adjustable see that they are set at the height that suits you best. Also, empty your grass box frequently; do not overload it.

Wheelbarrows

Very low handles make you bend down to pick them up. Do not try to wheel an overloaded barrow—extra journeys are better than pain. Whether you push or pull the barrow, carefully balance the weight and avoid twisting.

2. Problems at work

As work situations vary so much, you may not find exactly your job described here. Nevertheless, from the several different types of work that are discussed, there should be general principles that you can apply to your own situation to prevent pain arising from your work.

Office work

As an office worker you are likely to be sitting for much of the day and if you stay in one position for a long time this may produce back or neck pain. If pain does develop, you should have a change of activity and try to move around or take a walk.

It is vital to have the right office furniture. You should refer back to the section 'Sitting in comfort', as similar remarks about chairs apply to the work environment. Since we are all of different sizes and shapes, you need to work out for yourself what is the best arrangement of your desk and chair. If you have a very long back and you cannot alter the height of your desk, you may need to put your seat lower; if you are short, you may need to raise the seat. If you are really worried about your back or neck you must persuade your employer to buy some new furniture. You may find it helpful if your chair has a curved back (to support your spine) and is adjustable (so that your feet rest flat on the floor and your legs are flat against the seat).

If you are a keyboard or VDU operator, you may be at particular risk because you are likely to keep the same position for too long. Moving your machine might help. Screens should be adjusted so that your head is held straight when you are working.

It is now known that a telephonist may be at greater risk than almost any other office worker, because the strain of lifting a telephone directory at arm's length causes a considerable rise in pressure inside the intervertebral disc. To avoid this, telephonists should pull the directory near to their bodies before lifting it. Holding a telephone (and thus your head) at an angle can also create neck and back problems. If your job involves constant use of the telephone, ask your employer to provide you with a 'hands-free' headset.

Heavy industry

Surprisingly, those working in heavy industry are no more prone to developing back pain than anyone else. However, once a back problem is established it is likely to be worse and to keep you off work longer. If you have back trouble, talk to your personnel officer as well as your clinician.

Assembly line work

If you work on an assembly line you are more likely than others to develop back pain, although exactly why is not clear. Over the past 25 years a great deal of research has looked at working conditions, bench heights, and so on, trying to relate these to absenteeism for sickness—but few conclusions have been drawn. Again, if problems develop, talk to your personnel department as well as your clinician.

Farm work

There is no clear evidence as to whether farm work has an adverse effect on the back and neck or not. One could suppose that the farm worker of 50 years ago kept physically fit all the year round, whereas today's worker, bumping around on a tractor much of the time, is more likely to suffer from a bad back. But this is no more than an opinion.

Construction work

This is very variable but may well involve lifting and carrying heavy weights. If you are a bricklayer, you will know that two-thirds of your work is too high or too low for comfort, and mixing cement by hand is certainly tough on your back and neck. If you are a plumber or electrician much of your work will be in awkward positions.

Lorry drivers

If you drive a lorry you could be troubled by the vibration, heavy steering, and frequent gear changes. If these things cause you pain, pull into a lay-by, get out of the cab, and walk about for a minute or two. If your job involves loading and unloading then you have a whole new set of problems to think about. We give advice about lifting at the end of this chapter.

3. Travel

Public transport

You may spend much time standing at bus stops or on railway platforms. If sitting on a bus or a train you may find the vibration uncomfortable; see if things improve if you stand instead. If you do not have a seat, holding on to straps and jostling with your fellow passengers can also be sources of pain. All this is a matter of trial and error, and you may have to try to avoid travelling in busy periods.

Cars

Whilst driving you are sitting in one position for a long time. To minimize the risks of developing back and neck pain it is best not to lean the head and neck forwards, especially in poor visibility. A lumbar roll in the small of your back may be helpful. If you develop back or neck pain, stop and walk about for a while—don't press on.

Much has been written about the design of car seats. However, there can be no one perfect seat since the ideal angle of the car seat and the height of the head support will vary from person to person. You should bear this in mind when buying a car. Some people find that a beaded seat cover is helpful. The best positions for the steering wheel and wing mirrors are the ones that you find most comfortable. You may find that power steering and/or an automatic gearbox help you—so consider this when test driving new cars. Once again, all this can only be determined by trial and error.

Getting in and out of the car may hurt. When getting in, try sitting on the edge of the seat first, before swinging your legs in; swing your legs out before getting out of the car.

Loading and unloading the boot can also present risks. It may help if you keep your back straight and bend your knees, moving your feet rather than twisting your body.

Air travel

Take as little hand luggage as you can and divide it equally between both hands; struggling with baggage trolleys can be a source of pain. Plan as carefully as possible to reduce the time that you stand about in airports. If you do have a long wait, walk around. Seats in aircraft can cause back and neck pain so, particularly if your flight is a long one, it may be worthwhile trying to get a gangway seat so that you can more easily get up and walk about if need be. Inflatable neck rests (for sale in most airports) may also help.

4. Lifting—eight golden rules

1. Plan the lift. Do you need help?
2. Stand close to the object that you are about to lift.
3. Gain a good grip.
4. Secure your foothold.
5. Bend your knees.
6. Ensure that your back is straight.
7. Lift without jerking.
8. Once the object is lifted move your feet to put the object down. Do not twist or stoop.

5. Advice for neck pain

Collars

As with acute pain, a collar may help (although do not hesitate to abandon it if it does not).

Permanent or semi-permanent collars are available either from a hospital appliance department or from a commercial appliance maker; a permanent collar can only be obtained following referral by your doctor, usually to a rheumatologist or an orthopaedic surgeon. There is more chance of a successful outcome when the collar is individually fitted.

If you wear a collar all day you should be careful when driving or operating machinery and, especially, of going into a dark room from a light one. This is because the collar may distort some of the structures in your neck that control your balance and serious accidents can occur.

Pillows

Once more, you are the only judge as to whether these help or not. Many people who get neck pain in the evening find that a 'butterfly' pillow gives comfortable support, for example, when sitting in an armchair. (This is a pillow with the contents shaken out to the ends; the relatively empty centre is placed in the nape of the neck.) For sleeping, a down pillow (unlike a rubber pillow) will adapt to your shape and give you continuing support. How many pillows you use is entirely a matter of personal preference.

If you regularly have pain on waking, you should give thought to all this. A night collar might also be beneficial.

Posture

Many find that to hold the neck in a neutral position cuts down pain and discomfort. Stretching your neck as far as possible (the 'long' position) may also help, and is certainly worth a try.

Activities

With careful thought about activities, a great deal of neck pain can be reduced and avoided. The principles are as for back pain. Thus, do not maintain the same position for long periods, for example, when reading, sewing, driving, preparing food, and decorating; change activity the moment you feel discomfort. This is particularly important for keyboard and computer operators, who are very vulnerable to this kind of pain.

You need to plan your day, including activities that suit your particular pain 'pattern'. When carrying shopping or suitcases, the weight should be divided equally between both hands. Rest periods can be a good idea. If pain should start, do something different; just moving your neck may be enough. A collar may be useful when driving, but it clearly has to be soft enough for you to rotate your head easily. Be prepared to stop and walk around lay-bys as often as need be.

To reiterate, time spent planning how you can carry out as many activities as possible, is time well spent; you should aim to do as much as you can to help yourself.

Exercise

Appendix 1 includes an exercise that you may find helpful; you should however stop if it hurts.

Conclusion

Many people do not even realize how restricted their activities have become—so gradual a process it can be. However, having identified what has happened, the key thing is not to accept disability as an inevitable state. Having acknowledged that for self-help to be successful in reducing your disability, some pain and discomfort are necessary, you need to give some time and thought as to how best to gradually build up your range and level of activity.

To work at your disability progressively and systematically offers not only a chance of leading a life as near normal as possible, but will actually help reduce your pain. Adopting such a 'coping' rather than 'avoiding' attitude promises a much better outlook.

As each person is different, dogmatic instruction on self-help is impossible, but your clinician can give encouragement and general advice. The rest is up to you!

Key points

1. Because your case is inevitably individual, all your activities need to be thought about.

2. You need to assess just how disabled you have become.

3. If you want to improve your situation you must engage in increasing activity.

4. You may have to accept some pain and discomfort to achieve this.

5. If you do, you have a greater chance of leading as nearly normal a life as possible.

6. This should, of itself, produce some pain reduction.

7. All this is equally applicable to those suffering with neck pain.

12
Treatments that may help you

Introduction

We have seen that it is difficult both to find the cause of back or neck pain and to give an accurate diagnosis. This means that it is also difficult to plan treatment. Indeed treatment is often a matter of trial and error! It is important that you are aware of and consider all the available treatments, particularly if surgery is contemplated. There are many treatments on offer; the one you are given will depend largely on to whom you go for help. (The next chapter looks at the people who may help you.)

In this chapter we review 27 available treatments. Quite how they work, and indeed whether they will work for you (in either the short- or long-term), is largely speculative. So, if any particular therapy has failed to help you after three attempts, do not become downhearted; another treatment may well work for you. It's simply a case of 'back to the drawing board'.

Each treatment in this chapter is presented in the same way, usually answering the following questions:

1. How do you get the treatment?
2. Will the treatment help you?
3. Will the treatment hurt?
4. Can the treatment do any harm?

At the end of the chapter we give a quick and easy overview of all the treatments.

With regard to neck pain, all the treatments discussed (with the exception of epidural injections and rhizolysis and rhizotomy) can be considered.

Objectives

1. We discuss painkillers, anti-inflammatory drugs, antidepressants, narcotic drugs, and tranquillizers.
2. We review bed rest, heat and cold, electrical treatments, collars and corsets, traction, auto-suspension, and massage and manipulation.
3. We deal with local anaesthetic injections, steroid injections, epidural injections, trans-cutaneous nerve stimulation (TENS), acupuncture and acupressure, rhizolysis and rhizotomy, nerve root surgery, disc surgery, chemonucleolysis, and sclerosant therapy.
4. We survey hypnosis, biofeedback and relaxation response, behavioural therapy and cognitive behavioural therapy, and psychotherapy and counselling.
5. We give an overview of exercises.

1. Drug treatments

Analgesics (painkillers)

How do you get them?
Either over the counter or prescribed by your doctor. There are literally hundreds of easily available painkillers, including aspirin and para-cetamol.
Will they help you?
This will depend on the drug, the person, and the problem. Trial and error is the only way to find out what helps.
Can they do any harm?
All of them have potential dangers; many have unpleasant side-effects such as constipation. Also, we now know that taking pills can in fact make your problem worse. For all these reasons it is very important, if you suffer from chronic pain, that you only take painkillers when absolutely necessary. For acute pain, the policy is different and you will need to take full and regular doses of painkillers in order to do your exercise and activity 'programme' (see Chapter 8).

Anti-inflammatory drugs

As its name suggests, this class of drugs reduces inflammation and thus may help reduce your pain. Normally, they are available through your doctor, although Nurofen can be bought over the counter. The previous comments on analgesics apply equally to anti-inflammatory drugs for both acute and chronic pain.

If you have an ulcer or suffer indigestion do not take these drugs.

Antidepressants

How do you get them?
On prescription from your doctor. He or she will have good reasons for prescribing them and you must keep to the directions given.
Will they help you?
Ten per cent of patients seen at pain clinics are depressed and need antidepressant treatment, but there is little evidence to justify the much wider current use of them. Antidepressants should come low down on any list of treatments offered to you. On the other hand, in low doses they can relieve pain.
Can they do any harm?
Yes. They can have side effects such as blurring of vision and dry mouth. In such cases, contact your GP.

Narcotic drugs (morphine and its derivatives)

These are very strong painkillers.
How do you get them?
They will be prescribed by a doctor and used only when your pain is severe.
Will they help you?
Very likely yes; narcotic drugs are the most effective painkillers of all.
Can they do any harm?
Definitely yes; the risks of addiction are very serious. For this reason their supply is strictly controlled and doctors are reluctant to prescribe them. However bad your back or neck problem

may be, it is very dangerous for you to obtain these drugs on the open market.

Tranquillizers

These are widely prescribed today, often without good cause, and they share the same problems as antidepressants.

2. Physical treatments

Bed rest

How do you get it?
If you are immobilized with the pain, you will have no choice but to take bed rest. Do not worry about which type of mattress you should lie on—the important thing is to be comfortable.
Will it help you?
In a severe acute attack it may well be the only thing that you can do and it will certainly seem to help in the short-term.
Can it do any harm?
Yes. Bed rest for more than three days in an acute attack and two weeks with nerve root pain is regarded as harmful. The policy now is to stay out of bed if you can, unless the pain is unbearable (see Chapter 8).

Heat and cold

You may find the application of either heat or cold a help, provided you give enough time to either treatment. It should be applied directly to the painful area for at least 20 minutes and should be repeated at least once a day.

How do you get heat and cold treatments?
At home (using a hot water bottle or something from the fridge or freezer) or in a physiotherapy department.
Will they help you?
Quite likely, yes. They are certainly worth a try.
Will they hurt?
Not unless you overdo them and either burn yourself or get frostbite!

Electrical treatments

These include short wave diathermy (SWD), ultrasound, interferential therapy, and a number of other similar treatments.
How do you get them?
Usually from a physiotherapist, although others such as osteopaths, chiropractors, and those attached to sports clinics and fitness clubs do also use them.
Will they help you?
They may but there is no way of telling before-hand—again, it is a case of trial and error.
Will they hurt?
Only if wrongly used. You should certainly tell your clinician if you feel pain during the treatment.
Can they do any harm?
Again, only if incorrectly used. Since it is not known how these treatments work, they are less favoured by some doctors. (This is rather unfair because we do not know for sure how any treatment works.) In the right hands, electrical treatments are safe and sometimes successful. So they may well be worth a try.

Collars and corsets

How do you get them?
Usually on prescription, although there is nothing to stop you buying them direct from the suppliers; many types are available.
Will they help you?
They may. The only way to find out is to try them.
Will they hurt?
They should not but if they do take them off at once.
Can they do any harm?
Not much, but if they are not helping, you might do better to try another treatment. Somebody once said that the best collars and corsets should fall apart in three months—this would make people think about whether they had been doing any good.

Traction

This is a well-known treatment that is currently out of favour because it has not been shown to be better than any other. On the other hand, it certainly has its successes.
How do you get it?
Usually through referral by your doctor to a physiotherapist.
Will it help you?
Yes, quite often, but it is not possible to predict who will be helped.
Will it hurt?
It should not but if it does, tell the physiotherapist to stop.

Can it do any harm?
Not if you stop when it hurts! It is possible to give yourself traction at home using a simple apparatus. You may find this helpful but you should consult your doctor first.

Auto-suspension

How do you get it?
Preferably on the advice of your doctor, though you could buy a machine yourself.
Will it help you?
It may or may not; try it and see.
Will it hurt?
Possibly. If it does, stop using it at once.
Can it do you any harm?
Generally speaking the answer is no, if you stop when it hurts. Those machines that tip you up can cause discomfort.

Massage and manipulation

We group these two treatments together because they work in more or less the same way—in so far as they are understood. Manipulation is now regarded as a key treatment for acute and recurrent pain; it is also promoted, though of less value, for chronic and nerve root pain.
How do you get massage and manipulation?
The treatment can be provided by your doctor or he or she should refer you, in the early days of your problem, to a suitably qualified person such as an osteopath, chiropractor, trained physiotherapist, or medical manipulator. A massage can be given by a professional masseur, or by a friend

or partner. The use of aromatherapy oils with massage could be a pleasant experience and might help.

Will they help you?
Very often, yes. There is now a lot of evidence supporting the use of manipulation. Again, be sure that anyone treating you is properly qualified.

Will they hurt?
They should not. If they hurt more than a very little you should ask your clinician to stop.

Can they do any harm?
Damage from either massage or manipulation is very rare. However, if you have a 'numb bum' (a condition where there may be pressure on the nerves supplying the bladder) or become giddy when standing up or turning sharply, manipulation could be very dangerous for you. (Indeed, if you develop a 'numb bum' you should seek immediate medical attention.) There are a number of medical conditions that negate the use of manipulation—to be safe, get a properly qualified opinion. The only possible harm from massage is that, if it is very rough, it may produce bruising.

3. Injections, nerve stimulation, and surgery

Local anaesthetic injections

How do you get them?
Your doctor will administer them and possibly at many different sites, depending on the physical signs that are found during examination.

Will they help you?
Very likely, yes—although sometimes only in the short-term, as the effect may wear off after a few hours.
Will they hurt?
Any injection hurts but remember that the injection may help to get rid of a much greater pain.
Can they do any harm?
Not when given by a properly trained doctor.

Steroid (cortisone) injections

Steroids are often used with local anaesthetics, but they may be given on their own.

Similar remarks apply to steroid injections as to local anaesthetic injections. Many people are worried by them, probably because of media reports about the use of steroids by athletes and sportspeople. Be reassured that when used properly, these injections are often a great help and have very few and very minor side-effects. So, if you are told you should have one, you have no cause for alarm.

Epidural injections

There are two different types. The caudal epidural is given via your sacral hiatus (a hole in your sacrum, convenient for injection). This is a relatively simple procedure which can be carried out in the doctor's surgery. This epidural has the same problems and advantages as local anaesthetic injections. Lumbar epidurals can be very helpful but must only be given in hospital (often to women in labour).

There is currently a controversy as to whether Depo-Medrone (a steroid) should be used for epidural injections. If this concerns you and you are offered an epidural, you should ask what is in it. If you are still worried, do not have the epidural. Many doctors now use local anaesthetic alone because the results seem to be just as good.

Transcutaneous nerve stimulation (TENS)

So far as is known, this stimulation works in very much the same way as massage and manipulation.
How do you get it?
Usually through a doctor. However, you can buy a machine and administer TENS at home (after consulting your doctor). You may be able to have a machine on trial before purchasing one.
Will it help?
Quite likely. It is well worth trying if you have chronic pain.
Will it hurt?
No, unless you turn it up too high in which case it works as a form of hyperstimulation (as does acupuncture). It will still not do you any harm.

Acupuncture and acupressure

Acupuncture is the oriental method for relieving pain using fine needles inserted at specific points to stimulate nerve impulses. Acupressure does not use needles and can be practised at home; precise finger pressure is applied to the same spots where the acupuncturist inserts needles.

How do you get it?

Your doctor may suggest acupuncture, or provide it—though usually you will have to find an alternative practitioner. Many people offer acupuncture so make sure they have some sort of qualification and are experienced in its use. You can contact the Natural Medicine Society to find out about it and other complementary therapies. You would normally administer acupressure to yourself.

Will they help you?

Often yes, so they are well worth a try if other treatments have failed. Acupuncture is now well regarded in medical circles as it often helps and is so safe; it is particularly useful for chronic low back and neck pain.

Will they hurt?

Acupuncture may hurt a little; acupressure does not hurt at all.

Can they do any harm?

In the hands of an experienced, properly trained person acupuncture will do no harm. Try to check hygiene standards—all reputable practitioners will use sterile needles, discarded after use.

Orthodox medical scientists have now established that you can get substantial relief of pain from the insertion of an empty hypodermic needle into a suitable place. Although the placebo effect (when you get relief from something without medical properties because you believe you will get relief from the treatment) cannot be discounted, the results are better than could be expected from this alone. The only rational explanation is that every injection involves an element of acupuncture. So, if your doctor suggests this approach, give it a try.

Rhizolysis and rhizotomy

These are surgical procedures that involve killing some of the nerve endings.
How do you get them?
By referral by your doctor to a hospital specialist.
Will they help you?
They may.
Will they hurt?
Like all surgical procedures they may leave you feeling a bit sore.
Will they do any harm?
Not if given by a properly qualified person.

Nerve root surgery

This treatment is a last resort, when the pain has become unbearable and no way has been found to stop it. It involves surgery to cut the nerve supply to the offending part.
How do you get it?
By referral to a hospital specialist.
Will it help?
Often yes—since nerves are severed, pain messages cannot be transmitted along them to the brain.
Will it hurt?
All surgery involves some pain.
Will it do any harm?
It may do; all major surgery carries risks, which is why this should be regarded as a final option, not to be undertaken lightly.

Disc surgery

This is surgery to remove disc material which may be causing your pain. It has the same problems and potential risks as nerve root surgery and is similarly a major procedure which should never be undertaken lightly.

Chemonucleolysis

This is a rare treatment which aims to dissolve the nucleus pulposus. It consists of an injection, done under anaesthetic and X-ray control, into the middle of one of your intervertebral discs.
How do you get it?
By referral by your own doctor to one of the few doctors who administer this form of treatment.
Will it help you?
It may do. As yet not a great deal is known about the long-term results; arguments still rage as to how safe and effective it is.

Sclerosant therapy

This once widely-used treatment is currently out of fashion because it has no clear advantage over other treatments and is very painful. It involves the injection of an irritant solution to tighten up possible slack ligaments.

4. Hypnotherapy and psychological and behavioural therapies

Hypnosis

This has been much studied, particularly in the relief of dental pain where it has proved very useful. It has been found to be less valuable in relieving back pain, possibly because hypnotic suggestion cannot overcome a pain, the cause of which may not be known. However, it is still worth a try.

How do you get it?

Usually you will have to seek it out yourself, although your doctor may refer you to a hypnotherapist. Increasingly doctors administer this treatment themselves, for example, to help people give up smoking.

Anybody can offer hypnotherapy, so make sure your therapist is reputable; try to get some personal recommendations. In the light of recent scare stories about women being abused whilst hypnotized, it is worth asking your doctor to recommend another doctor who offers this service.

Will it help you?

Quite likely, but it is unpredictable.

Will it hurt?

No

Can it do any harm?

Yes; you may react violently to hypnosis. If you do (and no one can tell in advance whether you will), the situation must be handled by a properly trained, experienced therapist.

Biofeedback and relaxation response

These are psychological therapies, grouped together because they act in a similar way.

How do you get them?

Usually by referral from your doctor to a hospital. Either hospital staff will conduct the therapy, or you will be shown how to do it yourself, at home or as part of a class.

Will they help you?
They may help.
Will they hurt?
No
Can they do any harm?
No.

Behavioural therapy and cognitive behavioural therapy

Again, these two are grouped together because of their similarities; both involve counselling and are concerned with the psychological aspects of pain.
How do you get them?
By referral by your doctor to a hospital specialist.
Will they help?
Often, yes. They are particularly useful for those with severe chronic pain, and are intended to improve the quality of life rather than relieve the pain.

Psychotherapy and counselling

Psychotherapists and counsellors try to uncover any emotional causes of your pain, mainly through question and answer sessions. They may also help you to come to terms with your back and neck problem. (The relevant organizations are given in Appendix 3.)

5. Exercises

Exercise is the most likely physical treatment to be offered to you, although there is no evidence that it has a direct effect on the prevention or treatment of pain. Neither has it been proved that weak muscles increase your chances of developing back pain. It has been shown, how-ever, that exercises which involve a great deal of movement, such as touching your toes, can increase the pressure inside your discs, which may actually cause trouble. Perhaps, surprisingly, your stomach muscles can take some of the load off your spine; strengthening these therefore makes sense.

There are a lot of conflicting, uncollaborated opinions as to the value of exercise. Again, our advice to you would be to continue exercising if it seems to help—always remembering to avoid excessive movements. The key thing is to ensure that the exercises are safe to do. In the light of this we describe one back and one neck exercise that are safe and which you may find helpful (see Appendix 1).

Activities such as walking, swimming, and cycling are now actively encouraged (see Chapters 7 and 10), even in the face of pain (provided that it is not too severe), since there is evidence that they actually reduce your pain, cut down the likelihood of further recurrences, and help to keep you at work.

Conclusion

All of the treatments discussed in this chapter can help; all of them work some of the time, none of them work all of the time. Recent extensive evidence has led to some major changes of policy:

1. Bed rest is to be kept to the absolute minimum.

2. Manipulation is strongly promoted for both acute and chronic back and neck pain—particularly acute pain.

3. Activities, rather than specific exercises, are encouraged.

4. So too is active rehabilitation (that is, keeping active and at work if you possibly can).

5. You, and your positive attitude and hard work, are as important as your clinician in getting a result from your treatment.

Key points

1. All these treatments may help, so keep on trying.

2. Only consult those who are properly qualified (see Appendix 3).

3. If a treatment is painful, consider a change.

4. If a treatment is not helping after, say, three consultations, think about trying something else.

5. Cut down on bed rest if possible.

6. Consider manipulation—and consider it in the early days of your problem.

7. All these treatments, with the exception of low back surgery and injections, are relevant for neck pain.

Table 1 Summary of the treatments covered in this chapter

Treatment	How do you get it?	Will it help?	Will it hurt?	Will it harm?	Cost	Time
Analgesics	Chemist Doctor	Maybe … certainly in the relief of mild pain	No	Only if you fail to follow directions	A/B	A
Anti-inflammatory drugs	Doctor	Maybe … certainly in the relief of mild pain	No	Yes if you fail to follow directions	A/B	A
Antidepressants	Doctor	Maybe … but should be viewed with caution	No	Yes if you fail to follow directions	A/B	A
Narcotic drugs	Doctor	Maybe … but these are very strong	No	Yes if you become addicted	C	A
Tranquillizers	Doctor	Maybe … but should be viewed with caution	No	Yes if you fail to follow directions	A/B	A
Bedrest	Own steam	Maybe	No	No	Free	C

Table 1 (cont.)

Treatment	How do you get it?	Will it help?	Will it hurt?	Will it harm?	Cost	Time
Heat/cold therapy	Own steam Physiotherapist	Maybe	Yes if you overdo it and burn yourself or get frostbite	No	Free or A	B
Electrical treatments	Physiotherapist	Maybe	Yes if you overdo it	No	A/B	B
Collars and corsets	Own steam Doctor	Maybe	No	No	A/B	C
Traction	Physiotherapist	Maybe ... but out of fashion at present	Rarely	No	A/B	B
Auto-suspension	Own steam Doctor	Maybe ... but probably no better than ordinary traction	No	Possibly if you suffer from giddiness	A/B	B

					B/C	B/C
Massage and manipulation	Osteopaths Chiropractors Some doctors Some physiotherapists	Maybe	No—unless the clinician is very rough	Possibly, especially if you suffer from giddiness	B/C	
Local anaesthetic injections	Doctor	Maybe	Any injection hurts a little	Not if you are in good hands	A/B	A
Steroid injections	Doctor	Maybe	Any injection hurts a little	Not if you are in good hands	A/B	A
Epidural injections	Doctor	Maybe	Any injection hurts a little	Not if you are in good hands	A/B	A
TENS	Doctor Physiotherapist Own steam	Maybe	Rarely	Not if you are in good hands	A/B	A/B
Acupuncture	Doctor Acupuncturist	Maybe	Maybe	Not if you are in good hands	A/B	A/B
Acupressure	Self	Maybe	No		Free	B

Table 1 (cont.)

Treatment	How do you get it?	Will it help?	Will it hurt?	Will it harm?	Cost	Time
Rhizolysis and rhizotomy	Surgeon	Maybe	Yes	Not if you are in good hands	B	B
Nerve root surgery	Surgeon	Often	Yes	Rarely	C	C
Disc surgery	Surgeon	Often	Yes	Rarely	C	C
Chemonucleolysis	Surgeon	Maybe	Yes	Maybe	C	C
Sclerosant therapy	Doctor	Maybe	Yes	No	B	B
Hypnosis	Hypnotherapist —check reputable	Maybe	No	Maybe—if hypno-therapist not reputable	B	B
Biofeedback and relaxation response	Doctor	Maybe	No	No	B	B

Behavioural and cognitive behaviour therapies	Doctor	Often	No	No	A/B	C
Psychotherapy and counselling	Psychotherapist Counsellor	Maybe	No	No	B	B/C
Exercise	Self	Maybe	Not unless you overdo it	Not unless you overdo it	Free	C

In the cost column A = cheap, B = moderate, and C = expensive. The time column refers to how long the treatment takes to start having an effect: A = minutes, B = hours, and C = days or longer.

Conclusion

If you try any of these treatments and it fails to work, change it! Keep an open mind about treatments. Do not trust a dogmatic clinician.

13

People who may help you

Introduction

In this chapter we look at the different people who could treat your back or neck. In each case we try to answer some of the following questions:

1. How do you find your chosen clinician?
2. What sort of person will he or she be?
3. What will your clinician do to you?
4. Will it hurt you?
5. What risks will you run?

Many of the professions listed in this chapter have umbrella organizations (addresses of which are given in Appendix 3) to which any reputable practitioner will belong. They can advise you about the relevant complementary therapists in your area; your doctor will advise you about other orthodox practitioners that you may see. In addition, you can always contact the NBPA for information and advice.

Objectives

1. We discuss acupuncturists, Alexander technique teachers, back specialists, bone-setters, chiropractors, and doctors.
2. We review herbalists, homoeopaths, medical manipulators, neurosurgeons, orthopaedic surgeons, and osteopaths.
3. We describe pain clinics, physiotherapists, psychiatrists, psychologists, and counsellors.
4. We mention rheumatologists, sports coaches, and specialists in sports medicine.

1. Acupuncturists, Alexander technique teachers, bone and back specialists, and doctors

Acupuncturists

How do you get to one?
In almost every case you make an appointment on the recommendation of someone who has found acupuncture helpful.
What sort of person will they be?
Their training may be quite extensive and there are an increasing number of doctors practising acupuncture. However, there is nothing in law to stop anyone from setting up in practice as an acupuncturist. There is no generally accepted qualification and standards vary enormously, so be very careful when choosing one.

What will they do?
First, they will take a relevant history. Then, they will insert fine needles into your body, sometimes at points far away from your pain. They may leave them in for some time, occasionally giving them a twiddle. They may pass an electric current through the needles.

There is also a form of acupuncture called electroacupuncture in which no needles are used, but a current is passed through a blunt probe (electrode) placed lightly on your skin.

Will they hurt you?
They should not; if they do, tell them.

What risks do you run?
None, except for the possibility of an infection from an unsterile needle. Check the qualifications of your therapist with the relevant organization (see Appendix 3).

Alexander technique teachers

How do you get to a teacher?
Your doctor may recommend one or you can apply directly to the Society of Teachers of the Alexander Technique (STAT) for a list of teachers (see Appendix 3).

What sort of person will they be?
Teachers who have undertaken a three-year training course.

What will they do?
They will try to help you to help yourself. By hand contact and verbal instruction you are taught to avoid preparatory tightening before movement and, hopefully, to eliminate the harmful habits that often cause pain.

Will they hurt you?
No, nothing in the Alexander technique is hurtful.
What risks do you run?
Because of the nature of the technique and the training of the teachers, there is no risk.

Back and neck specialists

How do you get to a back and neck specialist?
By referral by your family doctor.
What sort of person will a back and neck specialist be?
Firstly, he or she will be a doctor. Rheumatologists and orthopaedic surgeons will have had a specialist training after qualifying in medicine. But back and neck problems are so common and disabling that doctors from widely differing branches of medicine come into contact with patients and manage their treatment. Thus, they too become specialists in neck and back problems. Who you see will be dependent on your family doctor.

Recently, firm guidelines, based on the best available evidence, have been issued as to how specialists should diagnose and manage neck and back problems. Reassuringly for the patient, these guidelines are so clear that there is likely to be little confusion as to how matters should be dealt with (see Chapter 16).
What will they do?
They will take a history and examine you; injections, manipulation, drugs, acupuncture, or hypnosis are all treatments they may consider.

Only a trained surgeon will operate on your back or neck.

Will they hurt you?

This depends on what they do; some treatments, for example injections, inevitably hurt a bit.

What risks do you run?

Because their qualifications demand a thorough training, these specialists pose as small a risk as any other well-qualified group.

Bone-setters

How do you get to a bone-setter?

In country areas you can find a bone-setter by word of mouth; they are rare in urban areas. Seeking treatment will be your decision alone since your doctor is very unlikely to recommend one. Bone-setters have no umbrella organization.

What sort of person will they be?

Bone-setters are unlikely to have had any formal training; the skills having most probably been learnt from a member of their family.

What will they do?

They will manipulate you—which may well help.

Will they hurt you?

They should not, but if they do, let them know straightaway. If a bone-setter tells you that the treatment is bound to hurt, do not wait for the treatment!

What risks do you run?

We have discussed the dangers of manipulation already. The rare disasters can be avoided only if the bone-setter knows how your body works and what can go wrong with it; this requires proper training.

Chiropractors

How do you get to a chiropractor?
Like osteopaths, chiropractors are now officially recognized. If doctors do not provide manipulation themselves, they are encouraged to refer patients to a chiropractor during the early stages of the problem. The British Chiropractic Association can recommend a properly qualified practitioner in your area; personal recommendation is another option.

What sort of person will a chiropractor be?
They should be formally trained and belong to a professional body such as the British Chiropractic Association. They concern themselves mostly with bone and joint problems and you may find that their treatment helps your back or neck pain.

What will they do?
In trying to make a diagnosis, a chiropractor will usually arrange for you to be X-rayed. However, it is now recommended that they modify their practice and reduce, by at least 50 per cent, the use they make of X-rays. In over 95 per cent of cases of back and neck pain, X-rays are of no help in making a diagnosis and, as they use high doses of radiation, they represent a danger.

The treatment they give is in general limited to massage and manipulation. They may speak of subluxation (when part of a joint has slipped) and adjustment (putting something back into place).

Will they hurt you?
They may. Some chiropractors use very considerable force (usually more than a osteopath will use) and this may hurt you.

What risks do you run?

If your chosen chiropractor is properly trained (see Appendix 3), the risks are minimal. The important thing is to choose very carefully who you go to.

Doctors (general practitioners)

How do you get to them?

Almost all of you will be registered with an NHS general practitioner (GP).

What sort of person will they be?

They will be one of over 30,000 in this country who will have been trained in a teaching hospital. After qualifying they will, by law, have had to undergo further training to become a GP. About a quarter of their work in general practice is to do with bones and joints but, unfortunately, their training in back and neck problems is inadequate. This situation must improve, and quickly, particularly since recent guidelines have put the emphasis on the handling of these problems in primary care. Doctors have either to intervene themselves in the active management of back or neck pain or refer to others to do so—and do this in the early days of the problem. What your doctor does or does not know about back and neck pain will become a more important factor.

What are they likely to do?

Usually they will prescribe painkillers and sometimes, other drugs. Your doctor should have due regard to possible side-effects from drugs and be able to explain to you what they might be. He or she may send you to bed. Bed rest should be restricted to a maximum of three days if possible; more than this can become a habit and actually make your problem worse. Your doctor may not be aware of this fact yet, in which case you should take the decision to avoid bed rest if you can.

Your doctor may arrange for an X-ray of your back or neck. Again it is worth repeating that in most cases X-rays do not help with the diagnosis, and indeed can be dangerous. In addition, your condition can become chronic during the time you have to wait to get the X-rays.

We discuss the circumstances under which your doctor is likely to refer you and to whom in Chapters 7 and 10. At present they are unlikely to use manipulation (although around 400 doctors do offer this treatment and this figure is likely to rise in view of the new guidelines). They are also unlikely to use hypnotherapy or acupuncture.

Will your doctor hurt you?
This depends on which of the many treatments available they choose; generally speaking they will not hurt you. If the recommended treatment is likely to involve pain, you will be warned.

What risks do you run?
Because of their training in general medicine, the risk of your doctor doing you a mischief is very small.

2. Herbalists, homoeopaths, manipulators, surgeons, and osteopaths

Herbalists

How do you get to a herbalist?
A register of medical herbalists is available on

application to the secretary of the National Institute of Medical Herbalists (see Appendix 3 for the address and telephone number). Most herbalists advertise in the Yellow Pages, but the best way is through personal recommendation. Look for the initials MNIMH or FNIMII after their name (both indicate that he or she is suitably qualified).

What sort of person will they be?

All members of the National Institute of Medical Herbalists have undergone a four-year training course.

What will a herbalist do?

The first consultation will last about one hour, during which past medical problems and family illnesses, as well as the present trouble, will be discussed. Any relevant psychological pressures will be considered when prescribing the herbal remedy. An examination of the back and possibly other joints will be carried out if necessary. Advice on diet and exercise will be given if required.

Will they hurt you?

No, but the medicine may taste unpleasant.

What risks do you run?

None.

Homoeopaths

How do you get to one?

The most common route is by recommendation; less satisfactory is to refer to the Yellow Pages. Look for the initials RS Hom. (registered member of the Society of Homoeopaths). The Society supplies a register of professional practitioners and the British Homoeopathic Association, one of doctors with varying levels of homoeopathic training (for addresses and telephone numbers see Appendix 3). Many health food shops and pharmacies carry details of local practitioners.

What sort of person will they be?

There are two main categories of homoeopathic practitioner. The first have undergone a formal training at a recognized college; the second are doctors who have done postgraduate training in homoeopathy.

What will they do?

A homoeopath will take a detailed case history in order to decide on the most appropriate prescription. Detailed information will be needed about current symptoms, past medical history, family medical history, overall level of health, and the present emotional state of the patient in order to establish how ill health is affecting the person. A homoeopath is less interested in commonly recognized symptoms and more in an individual's reaction to them.

As well as dispensing the relevant homoeopathic prescription (usually in tablet form), many homoeopaths will give general advice on relaxation techniques or changes in lifestyle that may be helpful.

Will they hurt you?

No.

What risks do you run?

Homoeopathic treatment can provide a safe and effective option for those who are in pain. If a homoeopathic prescription is inaccurate the most likely outcome is lack of response. Homoeopathy can be used to support other therapies such as osteopathy or chiropractice.

Medical manipulators

How do you get to them?
Bone-setters, chiropractors, and osteopaths all offer forms of manipulation. However, because they lack a formal medical training, none of these is a medical manipulator. Your family doctor may be one of the few hundred who use manipulation in the treatment of back and neck pain. If they are not, they may refer you to a colleague who does use it.

What will a medical manipulator do?
Doctors will, of course, be in a position to use other treatments if manipulation does not work.

Will they hurt you?
Medical manipulators should not hurt you. If they do, make sure you tell them.

What risks do you run?
Because of their training there will be no more risks than for any other doctor.

Orthopaedic surgeons

How do you get to them?
You are sent by your family doctor.

What sort of person will they be?
They will be a doctor who specializes in surgery on bones and joints, who has had at least eight years' training after graduating as a doctor. There are about seven or eight hundred of them in this country.

What will they do?
They will take a history and examine you, possibly ordering laboratory tests and probably

requesting X-rays. They often do their best to avoid an operation; they may use injections or manipulation. The decision to operate is not taken lightly. They will explain to you the advantages and disadvantages of surgery so that you can make an informed decision about whether you want to proceed with an operation.

Whilst orthopaedic surgeons, like rheumatologists, have been traditionally considered (by many doctors included) to be the specialists for handling back and neck problems, the fact is that many of them do not have a specific understanding of such problems. They often simply send you back to your doctor saying that you do not need surgery; your problem will be just as bad and indeed there is the risk that in the meantime your pain has become chronic. For this reason, referral to a pain clinic or a specific back and neck pain rehabilitation service is now recommended. This obviously makes sense, but it will be some time before these are set up country-wide. On the other hand an encouraging start has been made.

Will they hurt you?

They will not hurt you on examination, but if they decide on surgery you will have some pain.

What risks do you run?

All major surgery carries risks and therefore will not be offered lightly. Indeed, it will only be used if considered absolutely necessary.

Neurosurgeons

For the purposes of this book we can say that a neurosurgeon differs little from an orthopaedic surgeon. There are at present about fifty in this country. Their training is rigorous and they offer treatments very similar to those offered by orthopaedic surgeons.

Osteopaths

How do you get to them?
Ask your doctor, look in the Yellow Pages, or contact the osteopathic information service.
What sort of person will they be?
The osteopathic profession now has statutory regulation meaning that, in future, all osteopaths will meet the same standards of training and clinical practice, be covered by professional indemnity insurance, and adhere to a professional code of practice.
What will they do?
An osteopath will take a detailed case history and will want to know about the present problem and your previous medical history. He or she will examine not only the area which is painful but also other related parts of the body. The procedure is very similar to a conventional medical examination and, when necessary, osteopaths will request X-rays as part of the diagnostic procedure (although, for reasons already given (see chiropractors), their reliance on X-rays is likely to diminish).

Recent policy changes in how back and neck pain are managed mean that osteopaths, like other manipulators, will be given greater prominence.
Will they hurt you?
Osteopathy involves the use of predominantly gentle forms of manual treatment.

What risks do you run?
With a properly qualified osteopath, the risks are no more than for any other group of professional clinicians.

3. Pain clinics, physiotherapists, psychiatrists, psychologists, and counsellors

Pain clinics

These centres are relatively new and they bring together a range of specialists to advise patients on the management of chronic pain (including chronic back and neck pain). They aim to relieve the suffering of those with persistent pain, and to help those with chronic pain to live as near normally as possible, at home and at work. They are highly successful. Indeed, there is now to be a nationwide network of back pain rehabilitation services operating on the same principles as the pain clinics.

How do you get to them?
You are referred to a pain clinic by your family doctor or by a consultant.

Who will you see there?
They are usually run by a consultant anaesthetist because these people have a special interest in relieving pain and much experience of giving difficult injections. With the anaesthetist may be more doctors and also professionals from different backgrounds such as psychologists, counsellors, and physiotherapists. As mentioned before,

pain is dealt with by many medical specialities and it has both physical and mental elements. A pain clinic brings together various clinicians and specialists so that they can all contribute to fighting your pain and, above all, its effects on you. If you attend a pain clinic there is a high chance that you will be helped.

What will they do?

Those working in pain clinics may use any treatment that relieves your pain—including injections, acupuncture, and hypnosis—provided that it is safe. Patients whose pain they fail to cure will be taught how to live as fully as possible despite the pain; the results are very good.

Professionals in pain clinics also run educational courses in the management of pain for professionals from different fields.

Will they hurt you?

Whilst this depends on the treatment you receive, it is very unlikely that anything painful will be done to you in a pain clinic.

What risks do you run?

There are so many treatments you may be offered that some are bound to carry a limited risk.

Physiotherapists

How do you get to them?

Usually, your doctor will send you either straight to the physiotherapy department of your local hospital or, more likely, to a consultant neurosurgeon, orthopaedic surgeon, or rheumatologist. Any of these consultants may refer you to a physiotherapist. A number of physiotherapists practise privately; some in association with sports clubs. You may, of course, go directly to these or on the recommendation of your sports coach. In addition, many doctors now employ 'in-house' physiotherapists. The advantage for you is that you should be able to get an appointment much quicker than through a hospital.

What sort of person will a physiotherapist be?

They undertake a four-year basic training. There are over 30 000 in this country; roughly half of them deal with bone and joint rehabilitation (that is, helping you to get back to normal activity after a disabling illness). Whilst in the past they took instructions from doctors, they are now much more independent. It is likely that they will see you more often and be in a better position than other clinicians to note any change, altering your treatment as they think fit. If the painkillers your doctor prescribes do not work, you are quite likely to be referred to a physiotherapist.

What will a physiotherapist do?

They may use a number of treatments, each with its advantages and disadvantages; none of these treatments should hurt. The main therapies they use are:

1. Heat and cold—these are often used and are quite harmless if correctly applied.

2. Electrical treatments—for example, ultra-sound, short wave diathermy, and interferential therapy. The way these work is not fully understood but they are often helpful and are harmless, if used by properly trained staff.

3. Traction—again, no one knows quite how this works, but it is often successful and does no harm.

4. Massage—this is a good treatment and will often give you great comfort. It works in a similar way to manipulation but generally takes much longer to produce an effect.

5. Manipulation—a considerable number use manipulation of different types; you may find this helpful. Indeed, because manipulation is so actively promoted these days, more physiotherapists are likely to learn how to do it.

6. Exercises—your physiotherapist may ask you to perform a number of simple exercises on a regular basis.

All these treatments were discussed at greater length in the last chapter.

Physiotherapists are also key people in pain clinics and back pain rehabilitation services (see Chapter 10), where they set up graduated exercise programmes to help reduce the level of disability caused by pain. Available evidence proves that such exercise programmes work.

What risks do you run?

None, really, in the hands of a properly trained person. You also usually have the back up of the hospital if you are not making satisfactory progress.

Psychiatrists

How do you get to a psychiatrist?

Usually, you will have been referred by a consultant in another hospital department because your pain has not responded to treatments. There is now conclusive evidence that chronic pain always has a psychological side to it; so, if other people have failed to help you, the psychiatrist may succeed. As we have already said, when your back pain is not getting better, another form of treatment is always worth a try—provided it is safe.

What sort of person will they be?
After qualifying as a doctor, they will have spent many further years in studying the mind.

What will they do?
They will go into your history in great depth, looking for a psychological cause for your persistent pain. They will probably not examine or investigate you (as this will have been done in another department) but will either prescribe drugs or some form of psychotherapy. This aims to help you to come to terms with the cause of your pain through discussion; it can be very helpful.

What risks do you run?
A consultation with a psychiatrist carries no risk and will not hurt you.

Pain psychologists and counsellors

We discuss pain psychologists and their important role in pain clinics in Chapter 14 (which covers the management of chronic pain).

Counsellors tend to address very specific, easily identifiable problems. They are concerned with the mental or emotional components of pain and may or may not be medically qualified. You may find yourself one without referral from your doctor; they may work at pain clinics. The same remarks apply to them as to psychiatrists.

4. Rheumatologists and sports specialists

Rheumatologists

How do you get to them?
You are sent by your family doctor.
What sort of person will they be?
They will have had at least seven years' specialist training in rheumatic diseases after qualifying as a doctor. They do not perform any operations. There are only about 250 rheumatologists in this country; many NHS area health authorities do not have one at all. The shortage of funding in the NHS means that this situation is unlikely to improve.

Like orthopaedic surgeons, some rheumatologists do not have a specific understanding of back and neck pain. However, several are still involved in the setting up of the new back pain services which, because of the scale of the problem and the need to offer the widest range of treatments, draw doctors from many different medical backgrounds together. Our comments about orthopaedic surgeons apply equally to rheumatologists.
What will they do?
They will take a history and examine you. They will almost certainly order laboratory tests and X-rays to help determine the best drug to prescribe and whether or not you need some physiotherapy. They may give an injection or even manipulate you, but they are unlikely to prescribe any other form of treatment.
Will they hurt you?
This is very unlikely but if they do, tell them. There are little or no risks from a rheumatologist.

Sports coaches

How do you get to them?
Most sports and fitness clubs have a coach or somebody to administer immediate help if an injury does occur.

What sort of person will they be?
Almost anybody may be a sports coach. They may be an osteopath or a physiotherapist, but more likely they will have had little formal training.

What will they do?
Sports coaches give immediate treatment for injury which will vary considerably, depending on circumstances and training.

Will they hurt you?
They may; make sure you tell them if they do.

What risks do you run?
A sports coach may be the only person available to give you immediate help after a sports injury and in that respect you may have no choice but to do what they suggest. However, because their training can vary so much, you should be careful about accepting advice, particularly regarding exercise. Some of the exercises recommended may actually do you harm; a good sports coach is not necessarily an expert on backs! Standardized training of sports coaches would be reassuring.

Sports medicine specialists

How do you get to a sports medicine specialist?
By referral through your family doctor.

What sort of person will they be?
Usually they will be either an orthopaedic surgeon or a rheumatologist with a particular

interest in sports medicine; some may be doctors. What will they do?

They will take a history and examine you. They may send you for physiotherapy or give you an injection.

Will they hurt you?

They may—so tell them if they do! Because of their medical training, the risks are minimal.

Conclusion

As you can see, there are many people who can help you if you suffer from back or neck pain. We have described the functions of some of these people, and given you the information you will need to make a informed choice about your clinician and your treatment and to participate fully in discussion once a treatment has been prescribed. If you are being looked after by someone from one of the groups discussed in this chapter, but are making no progress, it is always worth asking for the treatment to be changed. If necessary, you may need to change your clinician.

Recent policy changes mean that physical therapists (osteopaths, chiropractors, manipulating physiotherapists, medical manipulators, and so on) are now strongly recommended in both acute and chronic back and neck pain.

Key points

1. Be prepared to try any of these people if your pain is not improving.

2. Ensure that whoever you see is properly qualified (see Appendix 3).

3. Be prepared to change your clinician if treatment is not working.

4. Bear in mind the new standing of the physical therapies.

5. All of the people discussed in this chapter could be as helpful (or not) to those suffering from neck pain as back pain.

14

Your consultation—the good, the bad, and how to prepare for it

Introduction

We have discussed a considerable number of people and treatments that you may come across. We will now give you some general ideas on how to detect whether your consultation is good or bad, whoever you are consulting. This is not only to ensure that you are getting the right help and advice but is also to prevent you being taken advantage of financially by the unscrupulous. We detail what should or should not happen to you, on the basis that forewarned is forearmed.

We know that patients remember only 40–80 per cent of what they are told in a consultation. This is not surprising given how stressful and worrying such an encounter can be for you. On the other hand, this is obviously wasteful and frustrating, so we describe ways to help you get the most out of each consultation.

Objectives

1. We discuss the history, examination, explanation, treatment received, and cost of the good consultation.

2. We do the same for the bad consultation.

3. We outline what useful information and personal questions you should have prepared.

4. We add some additional tips to help you get the most out of a consultation.

5. We explain why it may be helpful to take a friend with you.

6. We offer specific advice for those with neck pain.

1. The good consultation

The history

The person you consult needs to gain a full picture not only of your present problem but also of the sort of life you lead, your general health, and your previous medical history. No one can do this properly in a hurry. On each visit your history will need to be thoroughly updated so that if no progress is being made, the treatment may be changed accordingly. You should feel confident that the person helping you is prepared to spend time on your history and to seek clarification if necessary. You should also feel free to ask questions.

The examination

You should be prepared to undress to your underwear. The clinician will look at your posture and, to determine how far your movements are restricted and painful, will almost certainly ask you to bend forward, backward, and from side to side. He or she will also, as part of the same process, be looking for local numbness and test some of your reflexes, as these may indicate a nerve root problem.

Examination must be extensive and painstaking; this means that it will be time-consuming. Your whole spine must be examined and re-examined after every treatment to look for signs of change. Apart from what you tell the clinician about your symptoms, this is the only way he or she knows how the treatment is progressing. It allows them to decide on the next step. The examination must be repeated at every follow-up visit.

Your clinician may order some special investigations such as X-rays or blood tests, and these are discussed in Chapter 15. In a teaching hospital there may be medical students in attendance; if you do not feel comfortable about this, let your doctor know—the student can be asked to leave. Finally, be prepared for the fact that on the day of your appointment, you may have quite a long wait for your examination.

The explanation

Any consultation should include an explanation of what your clinician thinks is causing your pain, what they propose to do about it and answers to any questions you may have. Since a specific diagnosis is difficult to give, the explanation may not seem as clear-cut as you expect. However, the therapist who appears hesitant and thoughtful may well know more, be a safer person, and be more likely to change your treatment if necessary, than a colleague with a quick answer.

The treatment

The clinician who is prepared to change what they are doing if it is not succeeding knows more about your problem than the one who sticks to the same treatment whatever happens. After painkillers, manipulation is the most frequently used treatment for back or neck pain and should not hurt. You should make sure that any of the treatments you are offered is safe—ask if you are unsure of anything. If surgery is suggested, make sure your clinician spells out all the advantages and disadvantages, and do not be afraid to continue asking questions until everything is clear in your mind. If you want a second opinion, ask for one.

The cost

If you are paying for the treatment yourself, it is important that your clinician is able to give you a scale of charges and some indication of the total cost of your treatment. Be wary of those who cannot do this.

2. The bad consultation

The history

The consultation seems rushed, your chosen clinician skates over details that you think are important, and does not give you a chance to comment. Little or no history is taken; no proper history is sought at follow-up visits.

The examination

A sketchy and rapid examination is made that does not include the whole of your spine. No examination is made after treatment; no examination is made at follow-up visits.

The explanation

An overconfident and clear-cut diagnosis is given based on little history and a hurried examination. You should ask for an explanation of the diagnosis and why the treatment offered has been chosen.

The treatment

If the treatment hurts more than a very little, or the same treatment is given time after time without any real improvement, it strongly suggests that it is not suitable for you. The therapist may be rigidly sticking to his or her own particular interpretation of your problem. You should be wary if a long course of treatment is recommended in preference to therapy; there is more money to be made from the former!

The cost

Again, beware those practitioners who are unwilling to discuss costs or to indicate the size of the final bill.

3. Useful information and questions

It is worth spending a few minutes gathering useful information to take with you that will help the specialist. This should include, for the first consultation, an outline of your case history and details of any medicines that you are taking. At a follow-up consultation you will be asked about what has happened since your last visit and any side-effects of medication given to you. You also should have details of any dramatic change in your personal life such as promotion or pregnancy.

Questions are, of course, very individual but might include queries as to what treatment is being offered and why. If, on thinking back, you are not sure about anything that was said or done during your first consultation, compose a list of questions and make sure that these are answered on the second visit.

4. Some additional tips

From information gleaned from the NBPA helpline (see Chapters 16 and 17), we know what the most common concerns are that need addressing in a consultation. These include problems relating to the disability caused by the pain, anxieties about the actual condition, and worries about the diagnosis (which may not be as clear-cut as you would like). Make sure that you ask your questions. and get the answers. If you carefully prepare for each consultation, you should get the advice you seek from your clinician.

5. Taking a friend with you

This is often a good idea, particularly if you are worried and upset. Frequently a friend will remember something that was said that you had forgotten. They can also drive you home if you have had an injection; you can feel a bit shaky after such an experience.

6. Neck pain consultation

We emphasize that a consultation for neck pain should proceed in an identical way to one for back pain.

Conclusion

If you have any doubts that the people supposed to be helping you and the treatments they are offering are not doing you any good, or are not in your best interests, then ask questions. If you are not given satisfactory answers consider changing your clinician. If you choose to go to a complementary therapist, select someone who is a member of the relevant umbrella organization, if there is one. Addresses for these bodies can be found in Appendix 3.

You are likely to get much more out of any consultation if you spend some time writing down the information that the clinician is likely to want and the information that <u>you</u> want. A consultation with your doctor can be very variable and sometimes inadequate; you may not be examined at all. Your prepared lists of information and questions, and the presence of a friend, can be as relevant for a doctor's consultation as any other.

Key points

1. The good consultation is going to be thorough and unhurried, and will rarely involve a specific diagnosis.
2. The bad consultation will be the opposite.
3. If you are unhappy or getting nowhere with your treatment, be prepared to change your clinician.
4. Never consult anyone who is not recognized by their relevant bodies (see Appendix 3).
5. List the information you think will be needed and the questions you want to ask <u>before</u> you see anybody.
6. Take a friend with you if you think you need support.
7. The consultation for neck pain is identical to that for back pain.

15

Special investigations

Introduction

Special investigations are rarely needed or useful for mechanical pain. On the other hand, they are essential for an accurate diagnosis of potentially serious conditions. Blood tests and, particularly, X-rays are the most common investigations currently ordered by doctors. However, as we shall show, the number of routine X-rays taken is set to fall.

Objectives

1. We discuss X-rays—their dangers, irrelevance to mechanical pain and manipulation, their connection with chronic pain, and the need to reduce them.

2. We explain how 'wear and tear' shown on an X-ray is not, in most instances, related to your pain.

3. We review other tests such as myelography, magnetic resonance imaging (MRI), computerized tomography (CAT) scans, discography, and ultrasound.

4. We mention blood tests.

1. X-rays

The dangers

At present, three per cent of all X-rays are of the lumbar spine and they require 120 times the radiation dose of a chest X-ray. It is estimated that 19 deaths a year are related to spinal radiographs. The Royal College of Radiologists has recommended that the number of lumbar spinal X-rays should be halved.

Irrelevance to mechanical pain and manipulation

Acute mechanical pain is very rarely caused by conditions that show up on X-ray and there is no evidence that X-rays should be used before manipulation. In fact, doctors are now urged to order X-rays only if there is possible serious pathology or the pain has persisted for more than six weeks. However, at present they are still the most common form of investigation for spinal pain.

The connection with chronic pain

Not only are X-rays of no diagnostic help in many cases and, on occasions are even dangerous, but also, because of the delay often involved whilst you wait for an appointment, they can be factor in your pain becoming chronic.

Any clinician who orders a spinal X-ray may have the most excellent reasons, but you are fully entitled to ask what they are. Indeed, if a doctor thinks that you have a 'red flag' condition, they are advised not to get an X-ray taken but to refer you immediately to hospital since nothing may appear on an X-ray until the disease is quite advanced.

2. X-rays and 'wear and tear'

Many clinicians, including some doctors, believe that if an X-ray indicates 'wear and tear', then this is the cause of your back and neck pain and little or nothing can be done about it. However, this is not the case; there is no connection, in most cases, between such changes and pain, and no reason why you should have to 'learn to live with it'.

3. Other tests

Myelography

In this test, radio-opaque liquid is injected around your spinal cord in order to see whether the canal is narrow or if a disc is protruding and compressing a nerve root. The process necessitates a lumbar puncture in which a needle is inserted between two of your lumbar vertebrae whilst you lie on a table. This will be somewhat unpleasant for you. The table will also need to be raised and tilted in order to get a full view of what is going on—so be prepared for this as well. You will almost certainly be kept in hospital for 24 hours in case you get a rare reaction to the liquid or an unpleasant, but more common, headache. Happily, this test is used much less than it used to be.

Magnetic resonance imaging (MRI)

This is a more modern and improved equivalent of the myelogram that provides much fuller images of what is going on. The process does not involve injecting a liquid (nor the attendant headaches) but, instead, you lie within a magnetic field. Some people find the prospect of having to lie still for some time in a circular tunnel worrying or upsetting. If you do, you should say so.

This very costly technique is not available at all hospitals yet. Also, it cannot be used on people with pacemakers.

Computerized tomography (CAT) scans

These are an elaborate form of X-ray that again provide fuller information. It takes a bit longer to produce CAT scans than X-rays, but otherwise they present you with no problems.

Discography

This is similar to the myelogram and therefore involves an injection. On the other hand, because much less liquid is used, your body does not have to be tilted and you do not get a headache. The liquid is injected into the middle of the disc and there, if the disc is healthy, it stays. If the disc is degenerated it will spread and give some idea of the extent of the prolapse (hernia).

Ultrasound

In this completely painless technique, ultrasound waves are bounced off the spine allowing, again, a more complete image to be built up. These tests are particularly helpful in nerve root problems (less than five per cent of the total number of cases) since they provide fuller information about nerve root pressure. They can help to determine whether surgery is necessary and if so, what type of operation is required, and where.

4. Blood tests

These are of no value in mechanical pain. They are, however, particularly useful in identifying inflammatory 'red flags' such as ankylosing spondylitis and other conditions such as cancer. They will, of course, involve a needle in the arm.

Conclusion

Patients often ask for X-rays because they believe that they will help establish a diagnosis, so ensuring the correct treatment and increasing the chances of a cure. However, once they understand that X-rays are in most cases useless, can be dangerous, and may actually, because of the waiting time involved, make chronic pain more likely, they are then in favour of the recommendation that the use of X-rays should be much reduced.

All sorts of vital tests may be needed to sort out potentially serious problems. If you are concerned or anxious make sure you know exactly what is being done to you and why.

Key points

1. X-rays are of no use in most cases of mechanical pain.
2. They have their dangers.
3. During the time spent waiting for X-rays to be done, your pain can become chronic.
4. So, if you are offered an X-ray make sure you know why.
5. In most cases, there is no connection between 'wear and tear' shown on an X-ray and your pain.
6. Special investigations are rarely needed in mechanical pain.
7. They are essential for the 'red flags'.
8. All this is as true for neck pain as for back pain.

16

Helpline queries: the issues

Introduction

One of the services offered by the NBPA is a helpline which responds to your telephone queries and your letters. Over the years, much material has accumulated and this has been assessed by Myrad Kinloch. We are grateful to her and to the NBPA for allowing access to this information, which forms the basis of the statements in this and the next chapter. The information gives a clear picture of the main concerns you have (particularly with regard to chronic back and neck pain) and of the frequency with which these worries are raised. In many ways it is a record of your life with pain.

In this chapter we deal with the various issues in a general way; the next chapter focuses on your most common back and neck pain questions. Both chapters should be of interest to you and to your family.

Objectives

1. We comment on how important the issue of disability is to you.
2. We discuss the distress caused by confusion, worries about the family, your psychological state, and malingering.
3. We consider financial problems and the need for information (including useful addresses) on your rights and benefits.
4. We review questions about diagnosis, a cure, painkillers, and how long it will take you to recover.
5. We examine your dissatisfaction both with having been told to live with the pain and also with doctors and other advisers, and your need for reassurance and discussion.
6. We look at the situation with specific regard to neck pain.

1. Disability

You are likely to be much more concerned about the physical disability caused by your pain, and the effect it has on your life, than you are by the intensity of the pain itself.

Women frequently describe themselves as 'housebound' or say that they 'can't go anywhere any more'. Their inability to do housework is a problem; they worry that as a consequence of not being able to sit or stand for long periods, they may lose their job; and they are concerned that they might become physically dependent on those around them. Men are also concerned about housework and specific housebound activities; they worry less about general issues.

If disability is the greatest burden inflicted on you by your back and neck pain, it obviously needs addressing. Chapter 10 describes in some detail how successful multidisciplinary teams are tackling this problem. Unfortunately, not everyone has access to such teams. However, you could still adopt the techniques and principles they use, and Chapter 11 shows in detail how to do this. If a multidisciplinary team can achieve success in 85 per cent of cases, you should certainly be able to get some result.

2. Distress

Confusion

It is highly possible that you will feel perplexed, and in turn distressed, by the conflicting advice and diagnoses that you are given. Chapter 5 demonstrates how indeed this is a major problem.

A useful question

Any clinician dealing with a patient who is making little or no progress, would be advised to ask the question 'what have your friends or relatives been telling you in the last week?' In one actual example, the reply was that four other clinicians and five other forms of treatment (including surgery) had been suggested. Such a glut of contradictory advice can leave the patient feeling inevitably confused and upset. The clinician can help by taking the time to explain and clarify the problem; patients are often then much more able to cope with the pain.

Your family

You may well be concerned that family relationships might suffer as a result of your condition. Many women are anxious that they may become a 'burden' to their husbands; both men and women worry that family support and sympathy will be withdrawn if their pain persists. We have already shown in Chapter 10 how vital the family is in dealing with your chronic pain. However, the helpline queries show that often there is little discussion within the family about the problem and a lack of awareness about its implications for everyone. Nevertheless, it is very important to discuss the matter. After all, if the problem affects the whole family (and we know that it does), it makes sense to face it as a family.

Your psychological state

Disability, confusion, and your family are then the issues that upset and worry you most and that can leave you feeling anxious, depressed, angry, or guilty. It is hardly surprising that you would feel like this. As we explain in Chapter 9, chronic pain does have inevitable psychological consequences, including a 10 per cent incidence of depression. However, there is no evidence to suggest that those with back and neck pain suffer different psychological effects than those who have any other pain.

Malingering

The belief—and it is very common—that someone with back or neck pain is malingering is hard to explain; it seems to be part of our culture. There is no evidence, however, to support this view. Unfortunately, many of you, if asked by your clinician 'do you think you are putting this on or do you think I or your family think that you are putting it on?' would admit to some anxiety.

3. Financial disruption

A common type of query for the NBPA helpline concerns financial disruption. Patients are often worried that, if necessary, they do not have the funds to continue with 'alternative' treatments and, sadly, may have to take desperate measures to raise the money. In addition, they are deeply concerned that time off work can lead to reduced pay or even the loss of their job. Anybody who has to deal with people in this position can only be impressed by how they struggle, often under very difficult circumstances, to keep going. Such patients can hardly be termed malingerers!

Other queries to the helpline relate to information on rights and benefits. As the situation is both complicated and very individual, it is best to get expert advice; we detail how to do this in Appendix 2.

4. Clinical problems

Diagnosis

The CSAG guidelines have completely altered the situation with regard to diagnosis (see Chapter 5), and very much to your advantage. The profusion of diagnostic 'labels' can be ignored; 19 out of 20 of you will have 'simple' (that is, of a mechanical origin) back or neck pain. As unpleasant as the condition still is, a great deal of anxiety and distress is avoided if you are told that this, and nothing more dreadful, is the problem. The remainder of you will have problems which, if competently handled, can be quickly identified and managed.

A cure

Understandably many of you seek a cure. One of the most common questions asked of the people staffing the NBPA helpline is whether they know of a specialist who would be likely to help. In response to this, we would remind you that there are many treatments detailed in this book and, if you have not tried them all, it is worth doing so, since nobody can be sure of what might or might not work. If you have tried everything and you are still in pain then the chances of pain relief are relatively poor, but there is still a good possibility of reducing the level of disability caused by your pain (as we explained in Chapter 10). As we explained earlier in this chapter, disability concerns you probably more than the actual pain—and, in most cases, something can be done about that.

Painkillers

The use of painkillers for chronic pain gives rise to considerable concern amongst you. One problem is that many people take not only the tablets prescribed by their doctor, but also large quantities they have bought 'over the counter', with the resulting side-effects of constipation and frequently feeling unwell. You may worry about the possibility of becoming drug dependent—a justified anxiety because, as we have already mentioned, the more pills you take, the more this becomes part of your natural behaviour when in pain, and the less chance you have of reducing your disability. So, the more you can cut down on your use of painkillers, the better.

Recovery time and recurrence

Many people get very worried if their pain fails to clear or recurs. We now know, however, that back and neck pain recur more frequently than had been thought the case. Therefore, you should not consider a recurrence of pain to be either unusual or critical.

We discuss recovery rates in Chapter 6.

5. Dissatisfaction

Sadly, this is widespread; the majority of you will have been told that nothing wrong has been found with you and that, in whatever way, you must learn to live with your pain. Such advice—which surely promotes helplessness, despair, and, above all, passivity—is <u>absolutely</u> contrary to present-day information and teaching.

Whilst 53 per cent of those who contact the NBPA helpline regard the support from their doctor as satisfactory, the rest do not; a quarter are offered painkillers and no other treatment. Although 64 per cent are generally satisfied with 'alternative' therapies (14 per cent are not), 70 per cent would not ask their doctor for advice about these treatments. Thirty per cent would feel uncomfortable asking their doctor for a second opinion. All this suggests that communication between patients and doctors is not as good as it might be.

This situation is set to change however. The CSAG guidelines make it clear that doctors should address the concerns and worries of patients, and that more explanation and advice is needed. A Diploma in Primary Care Rheumatology for doctors has recently been set up, which includes specific study of the spine and is heavily influenced by the guidelines. Encouragingly, the first graduates to qualify claim that they now feel able to do far more for their patients with back and neck pain and, in addition, are themselves enjoying this type of work much more than before.

The CSAG guidelines also acknowledge that successful management of pain requires that the responsibility for recovery should be shared between the patient and the doctor. Progress can only properly be made with your help and commitment. This in turn depends on you having the information and advice you need. If you have concerns, problems, or queries you should voice them and get answers that satisfy you.

Conclusion

Your queries divide you broadly into three equal groups. The first comprises those whose principal concern is with diagnosis and cure. As we have noted, diagnosis should now be much less of a worry for you. As to a cure, when all else fails, emphasis should be on your reducing the level of your disability. The second group seeks more information, and books such as this are an attempt to meet this need. Finally, the third group requires personal assessment and discussion with a clinical adviser, whatever their title.

It is not surprising that there is widespread dissatisfaction at the present situation. Basically, those who suffer from back and neck pain feel that they need more time and attention. All are agreed as to what is wrong; all are determined to improve the situation.

Key points

1. Physical disability is your main concern, and it is the one for which most can be done.
2. The anxieties expressed with regard to chronic back and neck pain are perfectly natural; they reveal no evidence of neuroticism.

3. Worry about the possible lack of family support is very common and should be dealt with by discussion.

4. The vast majority of cases are of 'simple' back or neck pain; the diagnosis need not therefore be one of your concerns.

5. There is no evidence that you are malingering.

6. Most of you feel that you have been given inadequate advice and information, particularly by your doctor. The CSAG guidelines should remedy this for the future.

7. Many of you are concerned, and rightly, that you are taking too much medication. You should cut this down as far as possible.

8. For those suffering with neck pain, the position is exactly the same as for someone with back pain.

17

Helpline queries: specific questions and answers

Introduction

In the last chapter we considered the groups of problems that concern you most and how to set about tackling them. Here we discuss those specific back and neck questions that are most often asked. Some of the questions seek only further information; but in three quarters of cases advice is wanted. In a third of cases the problems are so individual that no book can give dogmatic answers. For example, with regard to surgery, each situation has to be assessed on its merits and you will have to rely essentially on your surgeon's experience and judgement. On the other hand we can direct you to where you can find the information you need and indicate how you should approach the problem.

Another feature is that each enquiry often has several elements that need sorting out. This is hardly surprising since back and neck pain frequently present many and sometimes inter-related problems. One thing is very clear, however, and that is that much of what we deal with here could and should have been discussed with your clinician. If you had prepared the questions that concern you (see Chapter 10), many would have been addressed.

Objectives

Back pain queries

1. We discuss the more common back pain 'labels'—disc bulge, degenerated discs, slipped discs, facetal arthritis, and sacro-iliac joint problems.
2. We deal with acute and recurrent pain.
3. We consider chronic pain, pain clinics, the back pain 'cure', recurrent pain on driving, and disability.
4. We look at posture as a cause of back pain.
5. We review the place of exercise and corsets and whether alternative treatments are available on the NHS.
6. We survey the problem of surgery.

Neck pain queries

1. We discuss the more common neck pain 'labels'—whiplash, cervical spondylosis, and ankylosing spondylitis.

2. We deal with acute and recurrent pain.

3. We consider the relationship between the neck and headaches, symptoms that are apparently caused by ear, nose, and throat problems, and the 'grating' neck.

4. We review chronic neck pain, neck pain and the computer, and travel.

5. We describe the role of exercises, collars, swimming, pillows, and beds.

6. We survey the problem of surgery.

Back pain queries

1. Back pain 'labels'

I have recently been diagnosed as having a disc bulge which is causing pain in the leg. Have you any information to help me cope?

In fact it is difficult to diagnose a disc bulge. If you do have one, then any pain it is causing will almost certainly be nerve root pressure which, as you can see in Chapter 5, has clearly defined features that you can check up on. Treatment for a disc bulge of recent onset is described in Chapter 7; what you yourself should do about it is covered in Chapter 8.

I have degenerated discs. What treatments are available?

Everybody has degenerated discs from early middle age onwards. On the other hand, not everybody has back pain and, in fact, you are less likely to get pain as you get older (see Chapter 3).

If they do cause pain it will be nerve root pressure, 'simple' backache, or, very occasionally indeed, as a 'red flag' (see Chapter 5). All too often, and incorrectly, this diagnosis is given as a cause of pain by even experienced and well-qualified clinicians. It seems that the professionals as well as the public need to be brought up to date with current thinking!

I have constant pain because of facetal arthrosis (degenerative changes of the facet joints). What does this mean?
In reality, very little. Exactly the same remarks apply in this situation as with degenerated discs.

A slipped disc that I have had for 18 years is causing me sciatica. Any advice please?
Discs do not slip. They can however prolapse (a form of hernia), in which case they can cause nerve root pressure (already discussed). If you have had pain for so long, we detail what to do in Chapters 10 and 11.

I have been told that I have a sacro-iliac problem. What does this mean?
Once again, this is a misleading diagnosis that does not mean much, but can be upsetting for you. The sacro-iliac joints can cause pain in ankylosing spondylitis (an inflammatory disease and a 'red flag' condition). However, this is rare, will be picked up by your doctor, and effectively treated. Most likely, we are talking about 'simple' backache. Without all this meaningless labelling, diagnosis and management of pain will be re-assuringly straightforward and effective.

2. Acute and recurrent pain

I have had back pain for a month and it is not getting any better. Should I do anything about it?

Indeed you should! This is quite a critical phase. You should seek help as a matter of urgency and proceed as described in Chapters 7 and 8. If your doctor will not refer you for physical therapy, refer yourself, but make sure you choose someone who is properly qualified.

I had back pain three months ago which cleared up. Now it's come back. I am very worried. Should I go to bed?

Do not be alarmed; this is really quite common (see Chapter 7). The management and self-help is the same as for acute back pain (see Chapters 7 and 8). You should certainly not take to your bed unless you have no choice, but should instead adopt a policy of maximum activity. Your slogan should be 'use it or you may lose it'.

3. Chronic pain, pain clinics, 'the cure', driving, and disability

I have had low back pain for 12 years including burning pain down the leg. What can I do?
The pain in my leg, which I have had for 10 years, is relentless. Any advice please?

Firstly, what treatments have you had? Read Chapter 12 on all the available treatments; consider those that you have not tried, because they might help. It is surprising sometimes just how little has been done. Too often we hear of patients who, having tried one or two types of painkillers with no result, have been told to learn to live with their pain, especially if an X-ray shows 'wear and tear' (see Chapter 15). This is absolutely the wrong advice and hopefully it will be given less and less by clinicians as they become more aware of the latest evidence. So, if there are treatments you have not tried, do so.

I am in constant pain. Can I be referred to a pain clinic?
If you have tried all the treatments then you should indeed be referred to a pain clinic or a back pain service using the same principles (see Chapter 10). In addition, you should give thought to the self-help advice in Chapter 16. What you do about chronic pain is every bit as important as what you do for acute pain.

I am looking for information about intensive rehabilitation programmes for chronic back pain sufferers.
This is covered in Chapter 10. Remember that the key word is 'rehabilitation'; you need to lead as near as normal a life as possible.

I have had back pain for 10 years. Have I no hope of finding a cure?
You may, but it is unlikely. On the other hand, pain clinics can often reduce your pain and, more importantly, can help you to cope a great deal better than you might have believed possible. You should not therefore regard the fact that complete pain relief may be as unlikely as the end of the world.

I get low back pain if I drive anywhere for more than 40 minutes. What can I do about it?
This is discussed in Chapter 11. Basically, it is a matter of planning. You should aim to split up your journeys as much as possible so that when you start to get your pain you can stop (perhaps in a lay-by) and do something else, for example, walk about for a minute or two. Do not press on; you will regret it if you do. You should also find out about different types of car seat, remembering that what is marvellous for one person can be torture for another. So, see if you can try some out before purchasing.

I find I am going out and doing less and less because of my back pain. Do you have any advice?
Yes, in Chapter 15. Your attitude to this problem is all important. Firstly, work out exactly what you are no longer doing—you may be surprised how much it is. Then set yourself a gradually increasing list of targets, to build up your activities. Start with what you know you can cope with, and add to it, bit by bit. Be prepared to put up with some pain; remember, 'hurt' does not mean 'harm'. Finally, take heart from the fact that very good results have been shown, time and again, to come from such efforts.

4. Posture

I am having increasing back problems. I have awful posture. I suspect that by compensating for the pain I am suffering, I am affecting other parts of my body. Advise me please.
Firstly, have you thought about all the available treatments? If so, and nothing has worked,

referral to a pain clinic or back pain service might be helpful. Many people worry about posture and are often given firm advice on the basis that it is all important. However, the fact is that there is no evidence to support this view. This is not to say that if you find, by experiment, that one position hurts and another does not, you should not act accordingly. Basically, you are your own best posture expert!

5. Exercise, corsets, and alternative treatments

I am a 36 year-old nurse recovering from a disc bulge. I would like any information or advice on how to get supple and what exercises are safe. I am wary of aerobic-type exercise, especially twisting and bending.

Firstly, you are absolutely right to think of getting supple; all the evidence points to the advantages of doing this. On the other hand, no one particular exercise has been shown to be especially helpful. We share your reservations about too much bending and twisting, as we know this puts added strain on the spine. The current position is to advise people to take such regular exercise as swimming, cycling, and best of all, walking, rather than using specific exercises. All these have been shown to be very helpful and to put minimal stress on the spine. Once again, set a gradually expanding programme of activity, and do not be too ambitious to begin with.

I have been prescribed a corset. What should I do?
Try it. Again, there is no evidence to show that these are helpful, but if it seems to work, then

fine. Alternatively, if it does not help or even makes things worse, be prepared to discard it.

What 'alternative' treatments am I entitled to on the NHS?
You are not specifically entitled to any. In the past, fund-holding doctors might refer you, for example, to an osteopath, but the cost for this would come out of their budget. Given their current financial pressures, they are far more likely to advise you to go to such a person and pay for it out of your own pocket (even though they are now being urged to make more referrals). This may change in the future.

6. Surgery

I have been offered a spinal fusion. Am I entitled to a second opinion?
If you are worried you can certainly ask for one. It might be better, however, if you discussed your concerns with your surgeon. He or she will understand your reluctance to embark on a major procedure without full discussion and thought. We cannot give you general advice because your case is so individual and only your personal surgeon will know all the details.

Neck pain queries

1. Neck pain 'labels'

I recently had a road traffic accident and following X-rays I was told that I had a whiplash injury and to go home and rest. What is it? What should I do?
Whiplash simply means a 'sprained' neck. Most

of the injuries settle down, heal, and cause no further trouble; some do not, possibly resulting in recurrent headaches, ringing in the ears, giddiness, and other symptoms suggesting an ear, nose, or throat problem. Unfortunately, many doctors are not aware of this and may even suggest that you are being neurotic. This is a pity as the right treatment can be very helpful.

As a general guide, wait at least two weeks before consulting anyone if you have the symptoms described. (Most clinicians would be reluctant to see you sooner than this because there is still time for the neck to heal of its own accord.) After two weeks you should see your family doctor who will treat you him or herself, or else refer you to an osteopath, chiropractor, or another doctor interested in these problems. A number of local treatments can be very helpful—notably manipulation, acupuncture, or, if need be, injections.

Three years ago I had an accident and suffered whiplash. Would an osteopath, chiropractor, or physio be able to help me after this length of time?
Very often, yes. It is true that the more long-standing the pain, the more difficult it is to relieve it, but in this situation the results are often very good indeed.

The results of a recent X-ray show that I have cervical spondylosis. Is it common? What does this mean and what can I do to prevent it worsening?
Cervical spondylosis is not only common—it is <u>universal</u> beyond early middle age. This is because it is simply 'wear and tear' and there is nothing you can do to prevent it worsening. It does not

necessarily result in neck pain and, in fact, fresh attacks of pain tend to be fewer in later life. In this it is exactly like the degenerative discs we discussed earlier in the chapter and, again, is a needlessly upsetting use of a diagnostic 'label'. It demonstrates how often neck problems mirror back troubles.

I have just received the diagnosis of ankylosing spondylitis in my spine, including my neck. Is this common? Please could you advise me on exercises and any self-help groups?

Ankylosing spondylitis is a 'red flag' and one of the conditions that your doctor should be screening you for. As a 'red flag' it is rare and usually you should be referred to a rheumatologist who, in turn, will probably want you to see a physiotherapist who specializes in exercises aimed at maintaining mobility (which is very important in this disease). It can affect the cervical spine, but much more commonly, the sacro-iliac joints and the lumbar spine. In fact, 75 per cent of cases present with low back pain.

Again, it is difficult to give general advice because this condition affects everybody in a different way. You need to address your questions to your clinicians; they can tailor the answers to your particular case. There is an excellent self-help organization called the National Ankylosing Spondylitis Society. Details can be found in Appendix 3.

2. Acute and recurrent pain

Two weeks ago I woke up with severe neck pain.

I have been taking Nurofen, but I am still in a lot of pain. What can I do?
You should take action now and get yourself to your doctor as soon as you can. After two weeks, active intervention in the form of manipulation is indicated, exactly as with low back pain (see Chapters 7 and 8).

I have had three attacks of neck pain in the last year. What is going on?
Almost certainly nothing. As with back pain, recurrence is quite frequent and more common than you might realize. Therefore do not be alarmed or despondent but, once more, ensure appropriate management and self-help.

3. Headaches, ear, nose, and throat problems, and the 'grating' neck

I suffer from recurrent headaches. My doctor says that I may have a neck problem. Have I?
For several months I have had dizziness and vertigo. Initially I was told that I may have a middle ear infection, but my friend says it could be problems with my neck. Could it?
The answer to both questions is yes, and we discuss this in detail in Chapter 4. It is important that you are aware that your symptoms are caused by a neck problem, because many doctors are not. Treatment of your neck in this situation is often helpful; if your doctor will not provide it, seek referral to someone else.

When I move my neck from side to side I hear a 'grating' sound. What is it?

This is a common thing which worries a lot of people. We do not know what is it but, happily, you can be reassured that it is nothing to be concerned about.

4. Chronic neck pain, computers, and travel

My son has had severe neck pain for the last six months and is now complaining of pain in both his legs. What treatment should he consider?
The symptoms mean that he needs 'screening' and he should be referred to a specialist to ensure that the problem is straightforward. An adequate diagnosis is necessary before embarking on any treatment. If he proves to have a 'red flag' he will be referred to a rheumatologist or an orthopaedic surgeon; if not, ideally to a pain clinic or back pain service as, after six months, he has chronic pain.

Could you please tell me how to cope with chronic neck pain?
We deal with specific neck problems in Chapter 11. As we discuss there, the principles are the same as for low back pain.

My work involves sitting at a computer for long periods. Please could you advise me about posture and positioning of the work station to alleviate the pain in my neck?
Posture and positioning of the work station are important, but general advice about these is difficult because individual circumstances can vary so much. Essentially, it is a matter of trial and error. However, it is well worthwhile

investing time and effort in this. The main advice in this situation is to plan your day, interspersing short periods of other activities that you can do when your neck starts to hurt.

Do you have any advice on travelling comfortably for someone with neck pain?
We deal with this in detail in Chapter 11. We would emphasize that time spent in planning is rarely wasted.

5. Exercise and aids

I have been told that swimming is a good exercise, but I notice that my neck aches after swimming. I can only do breast stroke. Is that the cause?
No one specific exercise has been found to be particularly helpful. On the other hand, we know that general 'exercise' (walking, swimming, cycling) is beneficial. The breast stroke is probably the culprit; we would suggest that you either learn another stroke or concentrate on, say, walking. A regular programme of exercise is a good idea (see Chapter 11).

What is the current thinking about collars for neck pain?
Exactly the same as for corsets; there is no strong evidence for or against their use. So, if you find that wearing one helps, fine; if it does not, do not persist. Collars can be uncomfortable in hot weather.

What sort of bed and pillow should I use to help relieve my neck pain?

Once again, it is all a matter of trial and error—but worth the effort! Do not buy a bed, or indeed any other piece of orthopaedic furniture, without trying it out thoroughly first. The NBPA will provide the names of companies who offer such furniture on a trial period.

6. Surgery

I have recently been referred to a neurosurgeon. I am on the waiting list for an MRI scan of my neck and I may need surgery. What are the pros and cons?
As with back surgery, this cannot be answered in a general way because each case is so different. However, no surgeon will embark on a major procedure lightly, particularly as surgical results are not that encouraging. Planning is very important; it is essential that you list all your questions and anxieties before you see the surgeon. He or she will be happy to discuss these with you as nobody wants to operate on someone who is confused or reluctant. Make sure you are clear about everything that is said.

Conclusion

As you can see, there are many similarities between the two groups of back and neck pain queries. The system of diagnosis, the management of both acute and chronic pain, and the treatments are almost the same in both; your approach to self-help in acute or chronic pain is virtually identical; and the same positive, almost aggressive, attitude is as necessary and yields the same dividends. The advice given to those suffering with back pain with regard to exercise, physical aids, and coping, for example, with travelling, gardening, or work, mirrors that given to those suffering with neck pain. Finally, a degree of scepticism about diagnostic 'labels' applies to both groups, and for the same reasons.

Much of the information and advice that you need should be provided by your clinicians. They are all busy people however, and doctors in particular are not going to spend time ensuring that you have fully understood everything that has been said. On the other hand, you can reduce your worry and confusion by coming to your consultation with your questions prepared beforehand (see Chapter 14); the clinician will answer your queries. In fact, because of the individual features of your case, the clinician may be the <u>only</u> person who can answer some of your questions.

Key points

1. The system of diagnosis for back and neck pain is the same.

2. So is the problem in relation to 'labels'.

3. So is the way acute and chronic pain are managed.

4. So is what you do in the way of self-help.

5. Time spent on planning your consultation and ensuring that you have understood what is going on will greatly reduce the queries you have and, therefore, your worry and anxiety.

18
Conclusion

The extraordinary explosion in the number of cases of back and neck pain shows no signs of abating. You have seen exactly how the pain can affect, and sometimes take over, your life—perhaps more than you realize. You now know the different problems that acute and chronic pain present for you and that there has been a radical change in thinking with regard to what should be done to you and what you should do yourself. In fact, things are moving so fast that a completely new review of the situation was undertaken barely two years after the previous one. This does not happen very often in medicine.

We can prove that if you do not have adequate information and actively co-operate with your clinician, you are likely to suffer more pain and lose more time at work than if you do. A positive, even aggressive, approach on your part is essential in managing both acute and chronic pain.

Your queries show how vital it is for you to prepare for your consultations and to persist in asking questions until you are quite clear about what is happening; regrettably, the clinicians will often be too short of time to volunteer this. Reviewing the hundreds of queries that come through the NBPA helpline, we are struck again and again by the fact that some of your worries could be greatly reduced just with more explanation. So, do not be afraid to ask.

Finally, if you suffer from neck pain, you are now in just as good a position to handle your pain as someone with back pain because the advice given and the attitude needed are the same.

Key points

1. The scale of the problem is growing at a massive rate.

2. Your experiences show how back and neck pain (acute and chronic) affect your life in all sorts of ways.

3. The new methods of diagnosis and management are so different that you need to know about them.

4. What you do if you have acute or chronic pain is also so different and important that you need to know about it.

5. You need to prepare to get the most out of each consultation and to make sure you understand what is going on.

6. Finally, the new methods of treatment and approach by patient and clinician have been shown, time and again, to produce results. If you are not aware of what is available, you cannot benefit from this new information.

Appendix 1
Safe back and neck exercises

As we have already pointed out, there is no evidence to show that any specific exercise is beneficial. Nevertheless, worldwide, exercise is the most common treatment currently prescribed for back and neck pain (although this is set to change) and many patients ask for advice about it. We know that some exercises, such as touching your toes or sit-ups, can actually put your back at risk. So, we describe two safe exercises which you may find helpful; if they hurt, then stop. On the other hand, it has been proved worthwhile to tolerate some discomfort when undertaking 'general' exercise such as walking.

A back exercise

Stand with your feet about 18 inches (50 cm) apart and with your toes turned in. Turn the palms of your hands to the front and then twist them round, forcing your thumbs backwards. At the same time tighten the muscles of your buttocks. Hold this position for about ten seconds, relax for five seconds, then repeat. You must do this exercise every morning and night, repeating it four times initially.

A neck exercise

Sit in a chair with your elbows apart and your palms, fingers intertwined, resting on your forehead. Maintaining your neck in a neutral position, press your forehead against your hands to tighten the muscles at the front of your neck. This should be isometric (that is, it should involve no movement of the neck). Start with two minutes a day and build up gradually to about five. As no movement is involved you run no risk and it should be painless.

Appendix 2
Your rights and benefits

Introduction

One of the principal problems that you may have, particularly since the Patients' Charter has introduced new regulations, is knowing what your rights are and what benefits you are entitled to. Many people suffering from back and neck pain feel that they need to know what their rights especially in relation to access to information and making complaints. The question of benefits raises different problems; the literature concerning this is extensive, complicated, and prone to change. We show you how best to tackle this difficult but very important area.

Objectives

1. We discuss the Patients' Charter.
2. We deal with the information issue.
3. We outline the complaints situation.
4. We review the benefits scene.

1. The Patients' Charter

The Charter has altered things a good deal, especially with regard to your rights and expectations. These, and other issues, are covered thoroughly in a pamphlet called 'The Patients' Charter and you' which you can get free by writing to FREEPOST, London SE99 7XU.

2. Information

To quote the aforementioned pamphlet, 'You have the RIGHT to have any proposed treatment, including any risks involved in that treatment and any alternatives, clearly explained to you before you decide whether to agree to it'. So you see, not only is it in your interests to know what is going on, it is your right.

If you want more information ring the Health Information Service, freephone 0800 665544.

3. Complaints

Again, to quote the pamphlet, 'you have a RIGHT to have your complaint investigated and to receive a full and prompt written reply'. Your local Community Health Council provides independent help and advice on making a complaint; their number is in the phone book. If you are not satisfied after a complaint has been investigated by the NHS, you can ask the Health Service Commissioner for England (sometimes known as the Ombudsman), who is completely independent of the NHS, to consider investigating your case. There are some matters which he cannot investigate; a leaflet explaining his powers is available. His address is Church House, Great Smith Street, London SW1P 3BW; tel. 0171 276 2035.

4. Benefits

We initially intended to produce a survey of the benefits scene in an effort to simplify things for you. Unfortunately, the situation is horrendously complicated. For example, in one publication, under the heading 'inability to work', there are the following subheadings 'incapacity for work, contributions and credits, statutory sick pay, incapacity benefit, transitional rules, and severe disablement allowance'. Similarly, under 'care and mobility' appear 'disability living allowance, attendance allowance, invalid care allowance, and help with mobility needs'. On the same page there are another 14 major headings, all with several subheadings. Obviously many of these are inter-related, but it is still impractical to give you an overview and indeed, because of the very particular problems relating to your own case, it might be misleading to give such generalizations. The area has been further complicated by the Disability Discrimination Act and Welfare to Work.

If you want information on benefits, the NBPA has a range of leaflets, publications, and videos that can assist you.

If you have, or think you have, a problem, you need expert advice. Every town has a Citizens' Advice Bureau and we suggest that you approach your local office. Other useful contacts are: Benefits Enquiry Line, freephone 0800 441144 and Disability Allowance, 1st Floor East, Universal House, 88-94 Wentworth Street, London E1 7SA (tel. 0171 247 8763). Do not try to tackle the problem alone; we know that appeals that are backed by expert advice are far more likely to succeed than an independent effort.

Conclusion

The Patients' Charter has altered things and if you want details, we have told you how to get them. The situation regarding benefits is so complex that you will need advice if you have a problem. With the right advice, you can often get more help for you and your family. So, do not give up!

Key points

1. If you want to know more about your rights and expectations, write off for 'The Patients' Charter and you'.
2. The situation with regard to information and complaints is quite clear.
3. If you have a problem in relation to benefits, go to your local Citizens' Advice Bureau.
4. If you have a problem, do not give up - get help!

Appendix 3
Useful addresses

Therapies

British Acupuncture Council
(Publishes a list of practitioners and a question
and answer booklet on acupuncture)
63 Jeddo Road, London W12 9HQ
Tel. 0181 735 0400

The British Association of Psychotherapists
(Will give information and advice if you are
considering psychotherapy)
37 Mapesbury Road, London NW2 4HJ
Tel. 0181 452 9823

British Chiropractic Association
Blagrave House, 17 Blagrave Street, Reading
RG1 1QB
Tel. 0118 950 5950

British College of Naturopathy and
Osteopathy
Frazer House, 6 Netherall Gardens, London
NW3 5RR
Tel. 0171 435 6464

The British Homoeopathic Association
(Will supply a register of doctors with varying
levels of homoeopathic training)
27a Devonshire Street, London W1N 1RJ
Tel. 0171 935 2163

British Federation of Massage Practitioners
78 Meadow Street, Preston, Lancashire
PR1 1TS
Tel. 01772 881063
British Medical Acupuncture Society
Newton House, Newton Lane, Whitley,
Warrington, Cheshire WA4 4JA
Tel. 01925 730 727
British Osteopathic Association
8-10 Boston Place, London NW1 6QH
Tel. 0171 262 5250
British Reflexology Association
Monks Orchard, Whitbourne, Worcestershire
WR6 5RB
Tel. 01886 821207
British School of Osteopathy
275 Borough High Street, London SE1 1JE
Tel. 0171 930 9254
Chartered Society of Physiotherapy
14 Bedford Row, London WC1R 4ED
Tel. 0171 242 1941
The Council for Complementary and
Alternative Medicine
(Will provide information on recognized
practitioners)
63 Jeddo Road, London W12 6HQ
Tel. 0181 735 0632
European School of Osteopathy
104 Tonbridge Road, Maidstone, Kent
ME16 8SL
Tel. 01622 685989
Fibromyalgia Association UK
PO Box 206, Stourbridge, West Midlands
DY9 8YL
Tel. 01384 820052

The General Council and Register of Naturopaths
Goswell House, 2 Goswell Road, Street, Somerset BA16 0JG
Tel. 01458 840072

General Council and Register of Osteopaths
56 London Street, Reading, Berkshire RG1 4SQ
Tel. 0118 957 6585

Institute of Complementary Medicine
PO Box 194, London SE16 1QZ

The International Federation of Aromatherapy
Stamford House, 2-4 Chiswick High Road, London W4 1TH

National Ankylosing Spondylitis Society (NASS)
3 Grosvenor Crescent, London SW17 7ER
Tel. 0171 235 9585

The National Institute of Medical Herbalists
(Will provide a list of registered medical herbalists)
56 Longbrook Street, Exeter, Devon EX4 6AH
Tel. 01392 426022

The Natural Medicine Society
Edith Lewis House, Ilkeston, Derbyshire DE7 8EJ

Osteopathic Information Service
Osteopathy House, 176 Tower Bridge Road, London SE1 3LU
Tel. 0171 357 6655

The Society of Homoeopaths
(Will supply a register of professional practitioners)
2 Artizan Road, Northampton NN1 4HU
Tel. 01604 621400

Society of Teachers of the Alexander
Technique
(Has a list of qualified teachers)
20 London House, 266 Fulham Road, London
SW10 9EL
Tel. 0171 351 0828

Support groups

Arachnoiditis Trust
623 Queens Drive, Stoneycroft, Liverpool
L13 5TZ
Tel 0151 259 0222
Arthritis Care
18 Stephenson Way, London NW1 2HD
Arthritis Care helpline, freephone 0800 289170
Other calls 0171 916 1500
The Disabled Living Foundation
380-384 Harrow Road, London W9 2HU
Tel. 0171 289 6111
Fibromyalgia Association
(Details of local fibromyalgia groups available)
Mrs Barbara Doodson, 8 Rochester Grove,
Hazel Grove, Stockport, Cheshire SK7 4TD
Helpline 0161 224 4811
Other calls 0161 483 3155
National Ankylosing Spondylitis Society
PO Box 179, Mayfield, East Sussex TN20 6ZL
Tel. 01435 873527
National Association for the Relief of Paget's
Disease
323 Manchester Road, Walkden, Worsley,
Manchester M28 3HH
Tel. 0161 799 4646

National Back Pain Association
16 Elmtree Road, Teddington, Middlesex
TW11 8ST
Tel. 0181 977 5474
National Osteoporosis Society
PO Box 10, Radstock, Bath BA3 3YB
Helpline 01761 472721
Other calls 01761 471771
Pain Concern
PO Box 318, Canterbury, Kent CT2 0DG
Tel. 01227 712183
Repetitive Strain Injury Association
380–384 Harrow Road, London W9 2HU
Tel. 0171 226 2000
Scoliosis Association UK
2 Ivebury Court, 325 Latimer Road, London
W10 6RA
Tel. 0181 964 5343
Spinal Injuries Association
76 St James' Lane, London N10 3DF
Helpline 0181 444 2121 ext. 229

Suppliers of back pain products

Anatomia Ltd (Back 2)
(Has a showroom and produces a mail order
catalogue)
28 Wigmore Street, London NW8 9OS
Tel. 0171 935 0351
The Back Shop
(Offers a mail order catalogue)
14 New Cavendish Street, London W1M 7LH
Tel. 0171 935 9120

Appendix 4
BackCare

In 1999, during its 30th anniversary, the National Back Pain Association launched its new name 'BackCare—the national organization for healthy backs'. It reflects our positive, dynamic and inclusive approach to back pain and healthy back care.

BackCare helps people manage and prevent back pain by providing advice, promoting self help, encouraging debate, and funding research into better back care.

We are the only national voluntary organization solely concerned with the needs of people with back pain, and offer them, their carers, and those who have a professional interest in promoting healthy backs:

Advice based on a multidisciplinary and impartial approach, reflecting current research evidence. We have a range of publications available, and also run a nurse-led helpline service.

Self-help through local branches that enable people with back pain to meet together, feel less isolated, discuss issues and approaches with a variety of speakers. Most branches organize a range of activities such as hydrotherapy, exercise, pain management groups, and loan of TENS machines.

Debate by identifying and raising the issues to help reduce the incidence and impact of back pain. We provide a key link with health professionals, government, employers, and trade unions, stimulating and contributing to debates for better back care.

Research funds to improve knowledge and practice in prevention and treatment. People with back pain want to know what works and what does not work.

You could help us to help you:

Become a member and receive our quarterly magazine to keep you up-to-date on thinking, ideas and experience of others. Access to our local branches and local activities. Special access to our helpline. Additional benefits apply to professional and corporate members.

Make a donation to help us fund further research, run the helpline for more hours, produce more specialist information, increase support for the self help branches, strengthen our voice for better back care.

Order information materials to ensure that you, your family, and friends are better informed on how to prevent or cope with back pain.

For further information, please contact:
BackCare
16 Elmtree Road, Teddington,
Middlesex TW11 8ST
Tel. 0181 977 5474
Fax. 0181 943 5318
E-Mail   back-pain@compuserve. com
Website   www.backcare.org.uk

Index

facetal arthrosis 181
family, involvement 85
family relationships 171
farm work 101–2
finance *see* costs of back pain

gardening 98–9
gender, and back pain 21
giddiness, diagnosis 31–2, 189

harm vs hurt 57, 76, 89
headaches 31
heat application 64, 113–14
helpline queries 168–77
  questions and answers 178–93
herbalists 139–40
history 155
homeopaths 140–1
hypnosis 122–3

information 159, 199
injections 117–22
interferential therapy 114
intervertebral disc
  bulge 180
  degeneration 180–1
  herniation 166
  prolapse 39, 181
  structure 8–11
  surgery 121–2

lateral canal 12
lifting 103
ligaments 13, 15
ligamentum flavum 15
local anaesthetics 117–18
lumbar vertebrae 7, 14
  referred pain 33

magnetic resonance imaging 165
malingering 22, 48, 172

management of back
    pain 53–60, 78–87
manipulation 64, 66, 67,
    116–17, 148
  CSAG recommendations 55–8
  medical manipulators 142
  urgency of treatment 182
massage 116–17, 148
mechanical pain, vs 'red flags' 40
medical manipulators 142
migraines 31
muscles, activity 15
myelography 164–5

narcotics 112–13
National Back Pain Association
    (NBPA) 2, 45
  helpline queries 168–77
    questions and answers
      178–93
neck exercise 197
neck pain
  activity 106
  and back pain 28, 43
  collars 68, 104–5
  ENT problems 189
  grating 189–90
  pillows 68–9, 105
  posture 105–6
neck sprain 32, 186–7
neck traction 115–16
nerve root pain 39–40
  bed rest 54–5, 59
nerve root surgery 121
neurosurgeons 143–4
nucleus pulposus
  chemonucleolysis 122
  intervertebral disc 9–10
'numb bum' 38, 62, 117

Ombudsman, *address* 199
orthopaedic surgeons 142–3
osteopathy 50, 144–5, 186

Index

Printed in the United States
61986LVS00001B/14

9 780192 630773